Child Language Development
Learning to Talk
Second Edition

Child Language Development Learning to Talk

Second Edition

Sandra Bochner PhD, MA, MEd

and

Jane Jones BA, DipEd

School of Education, Macquarie University,
Australia

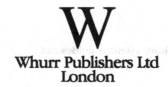

Whurr Publishers Ltd
London

© 2003 Whurr Publishers Ltd
First published 2003
by Whurr Publishers Ltd
19b Compton Terrace
London N1 2UN
England

British Library Cataloguing in Publication Data
A catalogue record for this book is available from the British Library.

ISBN 1 86156 379 5

Typeset by Adrian McLaughlin, a@microguides.net

Contents

Preface

Child Language Development: Learning to Talk Second Edition is concerned with the early stages of language acquisition. It is intended to be a practical guide that can be used by early childhood teachers, nursery nurses, special education teachers and others working with children who are experiencing difficulties in acquiring early communication skills. The programme described here is based on a developmental sequence that moves from the early skills of joint attention, turn-taking and appropriate play to the more complex skills of asking and answering questions. These procedures were initially presented in *Learning to Talk: A Programme for Helping Language-delayed Children Acquire Early Communication Skills* (Bochner, Price and Salamon, 1988) and *Child Language Development: Learning to Talk* (Bochner, Price and Jones, 1997). In this new edition, there is an expanded focus on the place of communicative intentions in early language development. Information on the use of augmentative and alternative communication to support early communicative efforts and on assisting children with language backgrounds other than English and children in group settings have been substantially revised and extended, and an additional chapter on working with families has been included.

The ideas presented in this and the earlier publications were strongly influenced by the theoretical work of McLean and Snyder-McLean (1978) and their transactional model of language acquisition. MacDonald and his associates at the Nisonger Center, Ohio State University modelled the translation of McLean and Snyder-McLean's theory into practice in *Ready, Set Go; Talk to Me* (Horstmeier and MacDonald, 1978). The contribution of these sources, together with the children and families who participated in the language programme of the Laurel House Early Language Group, and the funding support provided by the NSW Department of Aging, Disability and Home Care are acknowledged.

We are grateful for permission to reproduce selected signs from the book *Sign It and Say It: A Manual of New South Wales (Australian) Signs for Use with the Revised Makaton Vocabulary Adapted for Use in Australia at Stockton Hospital, NSW, for Communication with Intellectually Handicapped Residents* (Cooney and Knox, 1980).

Sandra Bochner
Bayview, Sydney, Australia
February, 2003

Introduction: Perspectives

This book is about language acquisition. Its specific focus is on young children who experience difficulties in early communication. Among the many skills that children must acquire during the first few years of life, language is one of the most important and the most difficult. Problems can be encountered as a result of a variety of factors. These include problems that the child brings to the learning task such as limited attention span, a hearing problem or difficulties in fine movement of lips and tongue. Also relevant are problems associated with the context in which the child is acquiring language, such as lack of opportunity to hear good language models or to take part in conversation-like exchanges with familiar adults.

Most children learn to talk in the years before school entry. However, a few experience difficulties and this can sometimes result in extreme frustration for both the children and their families. Children need to learn to communicate, to express their feelings, convey ideas and interact socially with others. Once they enter school, their language skills become the building blocks for literacy and numeracy. The early acquisition of appropriate language skills does not guarantee later success in learning at school (Paul, 2001; Fey, Catts and Larrivee, 1995). However, initial poor development is often difficult to overcome, putting the child 'at risk' for later problems in learning. So it is important to ensure that assistance is given as early as possible to children who are encountering difficulties in the early stages of language development, or to those known to be at risk for problems in language-related areas of learning.

Since the early 1970s there has been a dramatic increase in knowledge about the processes involved in children's acquisition of language. Much of this increase resulted from the work of psycholinguists such as Brown (1973), Nelson (1973), Bruner (1975) and Halliday (1975), who extended the work of linguists to explore cognitive, social and emotional aspects of the language acquisition process. These developments occurred at a time when McVicker Hunt had already challenged the notion that intelligence is fixed from birth (Hunt, 1961) and Bloom (1964) had documented the rapid rate of cognitive development during the early childhood years and the effect of experience on this process. Piaget (1962) had also emphasized the importance of the environment and the active role of the child in early cognitive development.

Recognition of the significance of early experience for children's subsequent development led to the concept of early compensatory education as a means of offsetting the impact of social and environmental disadvantage on children's progress at school (Chazan, Laing and Jackson, 1971). In England, local education authority nursery schools and classes provided programmes for some children from socially disadvantaged backgrounds. In the USA, Headstart programmes, introduced in 1964, provided compensatory educational experiences to socially disadvantaged, primarily inner-urban, black children in the period before school entry. From 1972, following recognition that children with disabilities would also benefit from these programmes, legislation was enacted which required that at least 10% of the children enrolled in these compensatory educational programmes should be handicapped. At about this time, early education programmes were also being established in the USA for groups of children with specific handicaps, including children with Down syndrome (Hayden and Dimitriev, 1975) and children with severe visual impairments (Fraiberg, Smith and Adelson, 1969). These programmes were characterized by a consistent, structured approach to teaching, with clearly defined objectives and parental involvement in planning and decision-making. They provided a model for exemplary early intervention services for children with disabilities, which were replicated in the United Kingdom, Canada, Australia and other countries (Pieterse, 1988). It was within this context that the language programme described in this book was developed.

About the language programme

The programme described here is derived from a theoretical model which assumes that early language skills are acquired through children's meaningful involvement with people, objects and events in their environment. According to this view, cognitive, social and linguistic aspects of children's experiences contribute to early language development. It is argued that 'first words' emerge out of children's earliest experiences with adults, particularly in situations that provide opportunities for infants to observe their carers' faces and listen to their voices. During daily routine activities and simple games, adults' facial expressions and the intonation of their voices encourage infant attention and engagement. Over time, infants learn both the actions and the sounds associated with daily routines and familiar games and, eventually, begin to take an active as well as a passive role in the social exchanges that are embedded in these events. These experiences provide children with opportunities to begin to produce sounds intentionally, to communicate specific, if primitive, meanings with familiar interactive partners. These are the contexts in which most children acquire language and they provide a model for the intervention ideas proposed here.

The language programme outlined in this book comprises a set of procedures that can be used to assess children's current language skills and, using this information, to design a series of activities and experiences that will increase their level of communicative competence. Teaching ideas are organized around a developmental sequence that moves from the prerequisite skills of taking part in a joint activity with a familiar adult to the more complex skills of asking and answering questions. Suggestions are made to help children progress through this sequence. Other related issues, such as the use of signing and the needs of children whose language backgrounds are other than English, are also explored.

How can the book be used

The book was written for use by early childhood teachers, nursery nurses, special education teachers, speech and language therapists, speech pathologists and other professionals working with young children with language difficulties. It may also be useful for parents of a child who is slow in acquiring language. It is suitable for use in initial training and professional development programmes in the areas of special education, early childhood education and care, and speech and language therapy or pathology. Procedures are described that are designed to facilitate the acquisition of early language and communication skills in young children with developmental delays and learning difficulties, either through direct intervention or by assisting parents who will implement suggested procedures at home.

Language-teaching activities can be carried out in one-to-one situations, with professionals working directly with individual children in clinical contexts, or indirectly, by supporting parents who implement intervention procedures at home. Programmes for individual children can also be implemented within group settings such as preschools and day care centres. In these contexts, language goals can be practised with children individually or within group activities where children can observe, imitate and interact with peers who can provide good language models.

Which children will benefit from the language programme?

The procedures described in the following chapters are designed for use with children who are not talking at a level appropriate for their age. The programme can be implemented with children who are having problems because of learning disabilities, developmental delay or intellectual impairment. Teaching ideas can be implemented using languages other than English. They should facilitate the acquisition of early communication and speech in children who have little or no expressive language, or who are just beginning to put two words together. The programme is *not* designed for children who have adequate language skills but are experiencing difficulties in specific aspects of language development such as pronunciation and morphology.

The approach to language development that underlies the procedures outlined in this book has been described as *interactional* or *transactional*. According to this view, children acquire language through interaction with familiar adults, usually their mothers or other consistent or primary carers. During such exchanges, adults provide clear models of appropriate language that children, in time, learn to first imitate and then use in meaningful ways. If the transactional view of language acquisition is accepted, failure to acquire early language skills reflects, at least in part, a failure to acquire the skills needed to interact successfully with others. This can result from two possible sources: factors within the social environment and factors within the child. Factors associated with the social environment may include:

- *Limited opportunity to participate in interactive exchanges with adults or mature language users.* The child's usual carer may be too busy or too preoccupied with other problems or responsibilities to provide the child with sufficient opportunities for interaction. Such opportunities occur most naturally during daily routines such as feeding, bathing and dressing.
- *Lack of consistent partners.* If the primary carer changes too often, the child may not have time to build up the set of interactive routines, shared with a familiar partner, that provide the basis for language acquisition.
- *Lack of recurring experiences with adults.* The child's daily routines may change too often, as when children are frequently moved from one setting to another, so that there is little continuity in their daily experiences.
- *Provision of poor language models.* These can include adult speech that is too complex or too fast, or where there is more than one language spoken. Many children do learn to talk in spite of such difficulties. However, the presence of other inhibiting factors may compound their difficulties and contribute to problems in acquiring appropriate language skills.

Factors within the child may include:

- *Lack of prerequisite skills needed to enable participation in relevant activities.* This may involve a very short attention span or an inability to attend to salient aspects of a situation. For example, a child may focus on a trivial part of a picture in a book, such as a leaf on a tree rather than the main topic which is a duck swimming in a pond.

- *Inability to initiate.* A child may not be aware that he or she can act independently or cause events to occur, or may not yet have developed a concept of self as 'me'. Once the child demonstrates the capacity to take both roles in a game such as 'Peek-a-boo', acting as either 'surpriser' or the more passive 'surprised', then you can assume that the concept of 'me' has been acquired.
- *The presence of a disability that interferes with the child's effective participation in social interaction.* This can include mild to severe or fluctuating sensory impairment (auditory and visual), restriction of movement arising from a physical handicap, or an intellectual disability.

About this book

The book comprises 15 chapters and, for convenience, is divided into three parts. Part 1 comprises the first four chapters and provides a background to the language-teaching ideas presented in later chapters of the book. In Chapter 1, the theoretical context in which the language programme was developed is reviewed. Chapter 2 gives an overview of the developmental sequence followed by most children as they acquire language skills. The language contexts in which children are engaged during the day is considered in Chapter 3, with both daily routines and play explored as important settings for language acquisition. The way adults talk with children is also very important in acquisition, and this is considered in Chapter 4.

The language programme is outlined in the chapters that make up Part 2 of the book. The first chapter in this section, Chapter 5, gives an overview of the steps to be followed in starting a language programme. The five levels of the language programme are described in Chapters 6–9. These chapters outline procedures that can be used to assess a child's current communication skills and to extend these skills through appropriate teaching strategies. Chapter 6 focuses on the preliminary skills that are the first steps in learning to talk (Programme Level 1). Chapter 7 looks at children's skills at the point when they begin to communicate, using gestures, sounds and made-up words in meaningful ways (Programme Level 2). The single-word stage is explored in Chapter 8 (Programme Level 3). Early sentences and the extension of meaning through the addition of morphemes are discussed in Chapter 9 (Programme Levels 4 and 5). Communicative intentions and the social use of language are considered in Chapter 10.

Part 3 contains the final six chapters. Children's phonological development or the production of speech sounds is reviewed in Chapter 11, and suggestions are made here for helping to improve the intelligibility of speech. For some children, consistent hand gestures or signing or other forms of augmentative communication can be used in the early stages of acquisition to supplement speech that is not readily intelligible. This issue is considered in Chapter 12.

Those who are helping children whose home language is other than English will be interested in Chapter 13. Issues that arise when a language programme is implemented in situations involving groups of children, such as a preschool, childcare centre or playgroup are explored in Chapter 14. Finally, Chapter 15 presents ideas for supporting families participating in the implementation of a programme designed to help a child who is having difficulties in developing effective communication and language skills.

The ideas presented in this book are based on experiences gained through a parent-based early intervention programme that was concerned with children who were experiencing problems in acquiring early language skills. The programme was implemented at home by parents who followed the suggestions made during weekly meetings with a special education-trained language teacher. Examples of the resource materials developed for use with parents attending the language programme, including information sheets, assessment protocols and record forms are appended.

Child Language Development: Learning to Talk is intended to be a practical guide for those seeking to help children who are experiencing difficulties in the early stages of language acquisition. It is not necessary to read all the chapters sequentially, although doing this will provide the clearest understanding of the language programme. Information about the theories that provide a background to the language teaching ideas suggested here are in Part 1 of the book (Chapters 1–3). Chapter 4, the final one in this part, is concerned with how adults talk to children. The issues raised here are particularly important and we urge all our readers to study this chapter.

Readers who are primarily interested in finding ways to help a particular child might focus on the chapters that comprise Part 2. Look at each of the chapters that describe the five levels of the language programme (Chapters 6–9) and decide the level that the child has reached. Some suggestions to help with this decision are included in Chapter 5. Readers who are uncertain should begin with Chapter 6, which is concerned with the early skills that underlie language acquisition. The skills described here are crucial for later development, so it is a good idea to check that the child can do the types of activities discussed in this chapter. Chapter 10 explores pragmatic aspects of language use: both the way children use their communication skills in the early stages of language acquisition, and the more complex uses of language. This chapter should be read in conjunction with Chapters 6–9.

Special education teachers, speech and language therapists or pathologists, and early childhood teachers or carers will be interested in all sections of the book. However, the chapters in Part 3 (Chapters 11–15) were written specifically for professionals involved in language intervention activities.

Part 1
Background to the language programme

The purpose of the four chapters in this first part of the book is to provide a general introduction to the theoretical ideas and research data that have influenced the ideas for language development presented in later chapters. In selecting goals and strategies for helping children to acquire early language skills, it is important to have some understanding of the explanations of language development that have influenced the work of others in this field. It is also important to have some knowledge of the results of relevant research. Since the 1960s there has been considerable expansion of interest, particularly among linguists, psychologists and educators, in the processes that underlie the emergence of speech in very young children. Much of the research that has been reported has focused on developing language in children whose communication skills are delayed or disordered in some way. Most children acquire language very rapidly. Data derived from studies of emerging communication skills in children whose development is less rapid are particularly useful because they provide researchers with opportunities to explore and begin to understand the factors, both within the child and in the surrounding environment, that facilitate language acquisition. Knowledge derived from these studies has been particularly useful for those wishing to help children experiencing difficulties in acquiring effective language skills. It was within this context that the language programme outlined in later parts of this book evolved. Issues related to the theoretical and research background of these intervention strategies are reviewed in the four chapters that follow here, as a prelude to the more practical ideas that follow.

Chapter 1
Explanations for language development in children

What is language? How do children learn to talk? Why do some children have difficulty in learning to use words? These are some of the issues that are discussed in this chapter.

Before you begin to help a young child to communicate more effectively, you need to know something about the term 'language' and the theories that have been proposed to explain its development.

What is language?

What is meant by the term 'language'? How does it relate to words like 'communication' and 'speech'? It is generally accepted that the term 'communication' refers to the process whereby information, ideas and messages are transmitted between people. In a very general sense, roads, cars and aeroplanes, as well as telephones, radio, television, books, newspapers and computers are part of our system of communication. Roadside signs and symbols such as a red cross, a church spire or a McDonald's big M communicate a message to those who understand the meaning of the symbol. A scream or cry of pain is usually understood by anyone who hears the sound. A touch or smile can also convey a message of sympathy or understanding. Communication in a very simple and direct form can occur without a formal language, without words. It involves the transfer of some message, or meaning, from one person or group of people to others.

Language is one form of communication. It involves an organized system of signs or symbols that are used by a group of people to share meaning. The signs or symbols can take the form of voiced sounds (speech), written symbols (text) or, for people with very poor hearing or vision, hand movements or raised dots as in sign language and Braille. Language in an oral form involves the use of speech.

All formal language systems, such as English, German, Mandarin or Hindi, have four main components:

3

- *Use* (pragmatics), function or purpose; what we want to do when we communicate. Some examples include uses to: attract attention ('look!'), obtain information ('how far?'), protest ('No. I don't want to!') or show ownership ('My ball!').
- *Meaning* (semantics) or the intended topic of communication. This may be represented in words (spoken or written) or through gestures, hand movements or symbols that represent the objects, events or experiences that we want to communicate about.
- *Rules* (syntax and morphology) or the grammatical system that defines ways of combining words to convey meaning. For example, the expression 'Mummy washed the red cup' is meaningful because the words are combined according to accepted rules, whereas 'cup red washed Mummy' is less clear because the words are not combined in an order that is grammatically correct. Meaning is also conveyed through the way a word is formed. For example, in English final consonants are added: to indicate plurality ('one hat: two hats'), to indicate possession ('the girl's ball'), to indicate tense ('the boy jumped').
- *Form* (phonology) or the mechanism by which intended meaning is conveyed to others. This may involve use of the voice to produce speech sounds, or a pen or pencil to write strings of letters to form words on paper. Alternatively, hand movements may be used to convey meaning through a sign language. For example, if a precise meaning is to be conveyed by both speech and writing, then a specific set of sounds (phonemes) and letters (graphemes) must be selected to go with that meaning, as in 'd'+'o'+'g' or [d] + [o] + [g] (Figure 1.1).

'd'+'o'+'g'

or   =

[d] + [o] + [g]

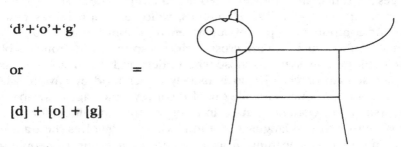

Figure 1.1

In planning a language programme for children, we need to take account of these four aspects of language. Initially, children must learn that they can communicate meaning to another person, using their own sounds, gestures and body language. For example, they need to understand that they can attract attention or obtain assistance to reach a toy by using sounds like 'oo-oo' or gestures such as pointing. Later, they will replace these primitive forms of communication with words. Once they have begun to use words intelligibly they will learn to combine these words according to the rules of their language group. When they reach this stage and can produce simple two- or three-word sentences it can be claimed that they have acquired the beginnings of a language system.

When thinking about the problems that a child is having in learning to talk, it is necessary to consider each of these aspects of language as a possible source of the difficulty. For example:

- *Use* (pragmatics). Has the child learned to use gestures, sounds, words, or body language to communicate specific meanings to others, such as to protest, obtain help or attract attention? (see Chapter 10).
- *Meaning* (semantics). Does the child understand that messages, including requests, comments and complaints, can be conveyed to others through voiced sounds, gestures, words and other means? (see Chapter 8).
- *Rules* (syntax and morphology). Are the child's words combined correctly to make meaningful sentences? Can the child modify words appropriately to indicate meanings such as tense, as in 'I fell down', or possession, as in 'Daddy's car'? (see Chapter 9).
- *Form* (phonology). Are the words intelligible? Are they produced in a form that can be understood by others? (see Chapter 12).

Examples of ways in which you can check each of these four aspects of a child's current communication skills are set out in later chapters of this book.

Explanations of language development

In order to help children acquire appropriate language skills, some understanding of the processes involved in learning to talk is needed. Ideas for intervention are likely to be most effective if they are based on a theory, or explanation, of how language develops and on information from relevant research. Various accounts of how children learn to talk have been proposed. These different explanations can be compared in terms of the relative weight that they give to two key aspects of the language acquisition process: first, the child's innate ability and second, the child's environment, particularly those aspects of the social environment that enable language to be acquired. These various explanations can be classified in terms of broad descriptive categories: for example,

- *nativist*, concerned with children's innate linguistic knowledge
- *behaviourist*, concerned with environmental influences or observable stimulus–response associations
- *cognitive*, concerned with the role of cognition or thinking processes in children's interaction with their environment
- *interactional* or transactional, focused on the place of social interaction in children's acquisition of language skills.

Each of these explanations is based on a different set of assumptions about how children learn to talk and why some children have difficulties. Moreover, each explanation leads to a different solution to the question of how to help a child who is having difficulties in some aspect of early communication. Nativist and cognitive explanations are mainly concerned with cognitive aspects of language acquisition, while the behavioural and interactional explanations concentrate on the role of contextual or social aspects of children's experiences in learning to talk.

Nativist or innate linguistic knowledge explanations

Some theorists (McNeill, 1970; Chomsky, 1986) have argued that learning to talk is a natural process involving an innate *language acquisition device*. According to this view, infants have an innate sensitivity to the sounds of language in that they are able to attend to and distinguish the way in which meaning is represented in the speech that they hear (Slobin, 1985; Cromer, 1991; Hirsh-Pasek and Golinkoff, 1996). This innate capacity enables them to achieve competence in basic grammatical relationships or the ways in which words can be classified and combined to create meaning. The concept of a language acquisition device helps to explain the remarkable achievements of children as they acquire language. Nativists argue that the primary task faced by children is to use their innate knowledge to learn the particular language that they hear being used around them; English, Danish or whatever is spoken at home.

At the time when the nativist argument was proposed, research into mother–infant interaction appeared to demonstrate that the speech directed to young children at home was degraded (disjointed and grammatically incomplete) and provided an inadequate language-learning model. It was assumed that children's very rapid acquisition of complex language skills during the first three or four years of life could not be explained simply on the basis of their exposure to language. A more satisfactory explanation assumed the existence of innate language structures that enabled children to learn the specific language system used around them. Evidence from cross-cultural studies of universal aspects of children's speech, such as the noun form, appeared to confirm the existence of an inborn predisposition for language. The fact that children are able to produce unique sentences that they could not previously have heard was used as further evidence to support the argument that children have an innate capacity for language.

Recent studies of early language development in children (see Howe, 1993, Snow, 1995; Dunn, 1999; Reznick, 1999) have raised questions about the adequacy of 'innate knowledge' explanations of language development. Although it may be acknowledged that children are born with an inherent capacity for language learning, it is argued that the process of language acquisition cannot be explained adequately by assumptions about innate capacities. Other clues from speech input are needed. For example, adults combine words with objects while interacting with infants (Tomasello, 1992; Hirsh-Pasek and Golinkoff, 1999). The increasing sophistication of children's perceptual skills (Slater, 2000) and their expanding cognitive and social abilities also contribute to the emergence of early language behaviour. More detailed studies of adults or older children interacting with infants have also demonstrated that although the language used in these exchanges differs from that used with peers, it is not degraded, as had previously been thought. Rather, it is finely tuned to the child's level in terms of simpler syntax and vocabulary, with higher pitch and exaggerated intonation in response to the child's vocalizations and smiles. Cross-cultural studies have also highlighted the significance of speech addressed to children in the language-acquisition process while challenging nativist claims about the existence of universal language mechanisms (Snow, 1995, p. 162).

Other criticisms of nativist explanations have focused on its negative view of the language potential of children with learning and other developmental difficulties on the basis that the problems experienced by such children are associated with limitations in innate abilities arising from the child's learning problems or disability. It must be acknowledged that biological factors contribute to language development. Certainly there is evidence that even newborn infants have an innate predisposition towards characteristics that are essentially human. For example, although the visual acuity of newborn babies is poor and they have difficulty detecting fine detail, their interest in moving stimuli and their skills in scanning faces develops quite rapidly (Slater, 2000). This is generally attributed to maturation of the visual cortex. At the same time, Locke (1993) argues that the helplessness of newborn infants, coupled with the length of time they remain helpless, ensures that they are placed in social situations which involve close contact and interaction with a consistent carer – in most cases, the mother. So early discrimination of the mother or primary carer's face, voice and smell may reflect the impact of *endogenous maturational processes* (Slater, 1989, p. 69). But studies of children reared in extreme isolation, such as the case of Genie (Curtiss, 1977) demonstrate that the acquisition of a language cannot be explained by maturation alone. Other factors also contribute to this process.

Behaviourist explanations

Behavioural explanations of language acquisition (e.g. Skinner, 1957; Mowrer, 1960), focus exclusively on the contribution of environmental aspects of the learner's experience. Language acquisition is explained in terms of observable phenomena. According to this view, children's behaviour is shaped by stimulus–response associations or the use of praise and rewards to encourage imitation and production of the sounds heard. Parents reinforce appropriate communicative behaviour, shaping the child's responses to achieve closer approximations to intelligible speech. Children are rewarded when they make speech-like sounds. According to Winitz (1969), acquisition of early communication skills begins when mothers vocalize during feeding. Following a classical conditioning model, the infant learns to associate these voiced sounds with feeding, a pleasurable event. The mother, in turn, is reinforced by the sounds made by her infant that seem, to her, to be an imitation of her own vocalizing. In this way, the sounds produced by both mother and infant become mutually reinforcing. This association is strengthened when the mother rewards the baby's vocalizations, particularly those that sound adult-like, such as 'mum-mum' and 'da-da'. These experiences encourage the child to further imitate adult speech models.

Behavioural explanations of language acquisition have a positive view of the potential of intervention programmes designed to assist children with learning difficulties and delays. As a result, behavioural techniques such as shaping, modelling, imitation and reinforcement, have been used to teach early language skills to children with learning difficulties and disabilities (e.g. Gray and Ryan, 1973; Kent, 1974; Stremel and Waryas, 1974). In general, these studies demonstrated that a behavioural approach could be used successfully to teach children to use new words. However, follow-up studies (see Garcia and DeHaven, 1974; Snyder, Lovitt and Smith, 1975) reported problems in generalization of the children's new language. For example, the children tended to use their new skills only when they were with the language teacher, rather than spontaneously when they were away from the training situation, either at home or playing with other children.

Overall, although behavioural models fail to adequately explain the complexities of normal language acquisition (Ward, 1997), techniques based on behavioural principles can be used to teach both expressive (uttering or using) and receptive (understanding or comprehending) language skills to children with delayed language. However, their use is limited. For example, behavioural techniques may not be effective in the very early stages of communication development when children need to learn that they can initiate contact with others. This is a particular problem with children whose difficulties are severe or profound in nature. Problems have also been encountered in ensuring the generalization of newly trained skills to settings outside the teaching situation. Behavioural techniques do, however, provide some very useful tools for helping children acquire early language skills. In particular, techniques such as modelling, imitation and reinforcement of desired behaviours can be used effectively in conjunction with other approaches, to facilitate acquisition of specific skills during regular language-practice sessions.

Cognitive explanations

The main issue addressed by those interested in cognitive explanations of language acquisition (e.g. Piaget, 1962; Werner and Kaplan, 1963; Vygotsky, 1986; Nelson, 1996) concerns the relationship between cognition and language. For example, does the child acquire the concept of an object before learning an appropriate label for that object? Or does the acquisition of specific words (such as 'gone') contribute, for example, to development of the concept of object permanence? Is the attainment of a specific level of cognitive development such as Piaget's stage 6 (object permanence) a prerequisite for the acquisition of words? Are some cognitive abilities, such as the transfer of information from one sensory modality to another, dependent on language? To what extent is intellectual development dependent on language?

Piaget's cognitive view of language development is similar, in many respects, to that of the nativists such as Chomsky (Ingram, 1989, p. 27; Cromer, 1991, p. 14). For example, both Piaget (1962) and Chomsky (1965) believed that linguistic knowledge gradually becomes available to the child through heredity and maturation. However, where Chomsky emphasized the significance of an inborn 'biological clock' in this development, Piaget placed much more emphasis on the contribution of maturation and, in particular, experience to the language acquisition process. Thus, whereas nativists believed that the processes underlying the development of linguistic knowledge were innate, cognitive theorists believed that the child had an active role to play in the development of cognitive structures. Maturation made more complex cognitive activities possible, but both cognitive development and language acquisition were the outcome of children's activity with objects, events and people in their immediate environment. The cognitive explanation of language acquisition suggests a very positive view of programmes designed to assist children experiencing difficulties in learning to talk, with clear implications for intervention involving manipulation of children's experiences within their social and physical worlds.

One of the issues that has concerned both practitioners and researchers in the field of language acquisition concerns identification of the developmental level or sensorimotor stage required for a child to begin to produce first words (Bloom, 1970; Brown, 1973; Ingram, 1978; Bates and Snyder, 1987). (The term 'sensorimotor' refers to the level of development reached by the child within the first of Piaget's stages of cognitive development, namely, the sensorimotor stage. This, in turn, is divided into six sub-stages that include 'means–ends', 'object permanence', 'goal-directed or intentional action' and 'deferred imitation' (Wadsworth, 1996). Early studies suggested that the attainment of means–ends (Piaget's sensorimotor stage 5) was critical. Scales such as those developed by Uzgiris and Hunt (1989) provided a tool to assess children's cognitive level as a basis for determining eligibility for a language programme.

Cognitively based research on early language acquisition has focused particularly on issues such as the relationship between the acquisition of a concept and related vocabulary. For example, does concept acquisition precede lexical development? Are new words 'mapped' on to existing concepts? Does the acquisition of a word facilitate concept learning, or is the word (a set of sounds that co-occur with instances of the concept) acquired as part of the concept? Can learning to read (recognize sound–symbol correspondence) be used to facilitate language development? Questions such as these have provided a trigger for a considerable body of research on the relationship between language and cognitive development (see Cromer, 1991; Barrett, 1995). In his review of the development of language and thought, Cromer (1991) concludes that general cognitive development is not an essential prerequisite for the acquisition of language, and that the two systems, cognitive and linguistic, develop in parallel, but independently. Shatz (1987) describes this as 'bootstrapping operations'. For example, children will begin to use a language phrase that has been heard but not fully understood. This contributes to their concept development by drawing their attention to aspects of their experience that had previously been unnoticed. In this way, development in one area facilitates or triggers progress in another. This view has influenced the development of procedures for facilitating early language development through use of strategies that map new language on to existing cognitive schemes or 'schemas' while at the same time using emerging vocabulary as a pointer for the selection and introduction of new concepts.

One of the main strengths of cognitive explanations of development is that it emphasizes the need for careful attention to be paid to children's developmental level, in terms of their progress through Piaget's stages of cognitive development. Children will extract meaning from their activities in terms of their current knowledge. The gap between what they know and do not know should not be too great. Children make sense of unfamiliar objects and experiences by mapping them on to what they already know and understand. Carers need to be aware of this and ensure that children can make a connection between existing knowledge and new experiences.

One of the main limitations of cognitive views of learning is that insufficient account is taken of the contribution of social aspects of children's experiences. Piaget described children as 'little scientists' in their exploration of the world around them. No attention is paid to the role of familiar adults who may be able to encourage and facilitate children's development by provision of both developmentally appropriate experiences and encouragement (or instruction) to assist in progression from one stage of cognitive development to the next. The cognitive view of children's development implies that there are limits in the contribution that carers can make to help children experiencing problems in acquiring language. Certainly, 'No amount of training will cause, say, a four-month-old to walk or talk' (Rutter and Rutter, 1992, p. 195). There is some evidence that children's cognitive development can be accelerated with appropriate instruction, though there is also evidence that they encounter greater difficulties in achieving these gains when compared with children who are left to progress at their own pace (Beilin, 1978). This has negative implications for the effectiveness of intervention with children experiencing problems in acquiring language. Piaget acknowledged the contribution of peer interaction to children's cognitive development, seeing such experiences as a means for children to expand their ideas and achieve shared solutions to problems that are more mature than those achieved by the children working alone (Brown, Metz and Campione, 1996). The role of adults is to provide appropriate activities for children as a context for learning.

Interactional explanations

It is now generally accepted that children learn to talk through interaction with familiar adults. According to this explanation, language skills are acquired as children take part in routine exchanges with the adults who care for them. This process begins from the time of birth, or perhaps, even earlier.

There is evidence that newborn infants have an innate predisposition towards other humans, which helps to ensure that they survive an extended period of extreme helplessness. For example, from the time of birth, infants appear to be attuned to visual stimuli, that are face-like – those with high contrast (dark–light) and involving patterns such as the eyes, mouth, and hair- and chin-line (Haith, 1980; Slater, 2000). Studies reported by Kaye (1982) have explored the feeding cycle of babies in terms of 'jiggle and suck' sequences; babies suck then pause, and during these breaks mothers tend to jiggle, stroke and talk to them. Debate about who controls the timing of this pattern of interaction has concluded that it is the baby, rather than the mother, as was initially thought. Clearly, babies appear to be 'pretuned' for social interaction, in terms of visual acuity and sensitivity to sounds, smells and touch. These issues are explored in more detail in Chapter 4.

Adult carers respond to infant signals of dependency and interpret these signals as communicative long before it can be claimed that the infant's actions are intentional and fully communicative. From the start, adults try to 'read' infant behaviour as if it conveyed meaning (hunger, discomfort and pain, pleasure, recognition). They respond to infants as if they were communicative partners from the age of 2 months (Schaffer, 1989), if not earlier. This behaviour provides a scaffold or language acquisition support system as proposed by Bruner (1983, 1999) and Vygotsky (1986: see also Lock et al., 1989) for the later emergence of intentional communicative behaviours and first words.

As children's awareness of objects increases, they begin to develop skills in integrating actions with both objects and people, using objects to attract attention and adults to obtain desired objects. Familiar action patterns are combined into more complex routines involving interactive partners. Bruner's descriptions of 'boo' and the 'disappearing clown' game (Bruner and Sherwood, 1976; Ratner and Bruner, 1978) are examples of this stage. Such routines, shared with a familiar carer, provide a very important first step in the development of language. According to Piaget (1962) it is through such recurring experiences that children develop 'schemas' or schemes (a mental image or collection of related ideas) that are used to organize existing knowledge about objects, events and people and make sense of new experiences.

Learning to play with a ball provides a good example of the way that children's 'schemas' for objects and events are developed. Children need to touch, smell, roll, drop and throw a ball to develop a concept of 'ball'. Part of this concept includes the sound of words that are used by familiar adults when playing with balls; for example, 'roll', 'push', 'kick', 'up', 'gone'. Most of this learning occurs when children play with balls regularly with a parent, sibling or other consistent partner. At such times there are opportunities to imitate what the other person says and does, to take turns in familiar routines and to practise new skills. Note that this explanation of language learning integrates physical, social and cognitive aspects of the child's experiences in acquiring language concepts. It also allows for some contribution from naturally occurring opportunities for imitation and reinforcement of appropriate behaviour by interactive partners. In a sense it combines aspects of all the views of language development described in this chapter. This approach assumes that all children can acquire the skills needed to enable them to communicate effectively with others.

According to the interactional view of language development, parents or other adults or older siblings can help children learn to talk by spending time with them, providing the children with opportunities to listen, watch, imitate and practise appropriate language skills. This model of language acquisition provides a particularly useful framework for developing an intervention programme that is based on parents, teachers or other familiar adults acting as agents of change for children with language difficulties. Using an interactional framework, adults can be taught to recognize both children's current level of communicative competence, and the contexts in which appropriate opportunities may arise to introduce and practise new language skills.

Criticisms of interactional explanations of language acquisition focus on the failure to acknowledge the possibility that there is an innate element in children's acquisition of language. Evidence to support such an assumption can be found in studies of children with pervasive developmental disorders (American Psychiatric Association, 1994) associated with problems in communication and socialization such as autism. These children's problems are neurological in origin and they usually experience extreme difficulty in learning and using a complex language system (Paul, 2001). Another problem arises from the assumption that children's acquisition of more complex aspects of their language system can be explained in terms of their daily interactive experiences with mature language users. If words are directly mapped on to elements of children's cognitive and social experiences, it could be predicted that the order of word acquisition would be universal across languages, and clearly this is not so (Hirsh-Pasek and Golinkoff, 1999). Language learning is a complex process. Interactive explanations provide a practical framework for understanding the initial stages of language acquisition, but cognitive processes are also involved.

The ideas set out in the remaining chapters of this book for teaching language to children whose acquisition is delayed are strongly influenced by interactional and cognitive explanations for language learning. These include McLean and Snyder-McLean (1978) in their review of language teaching strategies for children with disabilities and delays, and psycholinguists and psychologists such as Bruner (1975), Bates (1976), Greenfield and Smith (1976), Dore (1978) and Halliday (1975). Theoretical accounts of early symbolic behaviour by Piaget (1962), Werner and Kaplan (1963) and Vygotsky (Bodrova and Leong, 1996), and speech act theory outlined by Austin (1962) and Searle (1969) are also relevant. These various sources emphasize the significance of cognitive development, socially interactive experiences and the emergence of communicative behaviour in the acquisition of early language skills. Useful reviews can be found in Ingram (1989), Locke (1993), Gallaway and Richards (1994), Fletcher and MacWhinney (1995) and Zelazo, Astington and Olsen (1999).

Summary

In this chapter, the meaning of words such as 'communication', 'language' and 'speech' are defined. Some of the theoretical explanations of the processes involved in language acquisition are considered. These include ideas involving innate knowledge (nativist explanations), imitation, modelling and reinforcement (behavioural explanations), concept development (cognitive explanations) and social interaction (interactional or transactional explanations). The implications of each of these theoretical approaches to the difficulties faced by some children in learning to talk are considered. It is concluded that the interactional and cognitive explanations, focusing on the role of parents, teachers and other interactive partners, coupled with the active role of the child, provide the most useful model for helping children learn to communicate more effectively.

The next chapter will describe the developmental levels that children pass through as they learn to communicate as a basis for understanding how children begin to talk.

Chapter 2
Acquiring language:
the developmental sequence

In this chapter, the sequences that children pass through as they learn to talk are described. These sequences provide a framework for the language programme set out in Part 2 of this book.

How does language develop?

The process of language acquisition is often described in terms of a continuum or process of gradual change. It begins soon after birth at a point that precedes intentional communication and continues to the level where children are able to use language in more complex ways, such as asking questions and indicating plurality. However, this process does not always proceed evenly. There are often growth spurts, when change is very rapid, as well as plateaus, when progress seems to slow and little change in skills is evident.

Language development is also frequently described in terms of a sequential set of milestones, steps or stages of achievement, such as the 'preverbal' stage or the 'single-word' stage. These labels refer to a cluster of related behaviours that tend to occur together as children begin to communicate. For example, children often begin to use both consistent sounds and gestures in the preverbal stage. Later, in the single-word stage, they begin to label objects, actions and people. Ages are often attached to these stages, which can then be described as a 'developmental calendar' (Kent and Miolo, 1995).

Various models of the stages in language development have been proposed. For example, Ingram (1989, p. 53) identifies five major periods in the language acquisition process based on detailed descriptions of emerging child language by three linguists: Stern (1924), Nice (1925) and Brown (1973). An alternative model, based on Piaget's six stages in the sensorimotor period, is presented by Goldbart (1988, p. 23). In each case, it is assumed that individual children will progress through each level in the predicted sequence, with a gradual transition from one to the next as current skills are replaced by more complex behaviours. Patterns of development may also be uneven, with some aspects of behaviour progressing more rapidly than others; for example, receptive skills often appear before equivalent expressive skills. Moreover, once a child has reached a specific stage, such as the use of single words, development may appear to slow down. Occasionally, some form of intervention or change in the child's social environment may be needed to stimulate further progress. Overall, the concept of levels of development provides a convenient way to talk about the sequence of steps that are associated with children's language development, as in 'Josh is at the single-word level'. Ingram (1989) has a detailed discussion of this topic.

Other sources of information about the sequence of skills that emerge as language develops include studies of early language in small samples of children, such as those reported by Bloom (1970), Brown (1973), Halliday (1975; 1979) and Bates (1976). Useful data can also be found in large-scale surveys of emerging language skills in children who are developing normally. Information of this latter type is often reported in standardized tests of child development that cover aspects of language, such as Knobloch, Stevens and Malone (1980), Uzgiris and Hunt (1989) and Harrison et al. (1990). Standardized tests of child language such as those of Boehm (1986), Kiernan and Reid (1987), Pond, Steiner and Zimmerman (1992) or Hedrick, Prather and Tobin (1995) include similar information. The model proposed below is based on data derived from these various sources.

Levels in language development

The language programme described in this volume covers the levels that can be observed in the period described at the beginning of this chapter. It starts with the preliminary skills that precede the emergence of first words and continues to the point where the child can demonstrate acquisition of the more complex language skills acquired by most children in the years before school entry. The first level of the programme is concerned with skills that emerge when the infant begins to use consonants in vocalizations (Sapp, 2001), attend to objects and events as well as people, and use objects appropriately – not just mouthing or holding them. This is sometimes described as Piaget's sensorimotor stage 3 (see Goldbart, 1988, p. 23).

From birth, carers attribute meaning to infants by 'interpreting' their behaviours. However, as infants gain increasing control over their actions and interactions with others, it becomes obvious that they can now use consistent sounds, gestures or movements intentionally to convey meaning. They are beginning to acquire competence in the pragmatic aspect of communication. This is the point where the language programme begins.

The first level of the programme is concerned with developing skills that are considered to be prerequisites for language. There are three categories of related skills here:

- *looking together:* joint attention or the ability to look at something of interest with a partner, to follow their gaze and look at what they are observing
- *turn-taking and imitation:* the ability to interact with a partner and copy the partner's actions and vocalizations
- *appropriate play:* the ability to play in a commonly accepted way with a variety of familiar objects; for example, by shaking, putting in, dropping, waving, pulling and pushing an object rather than just holding or mouthing it.

The programme continues to the level where single words are combined into more complex utterances, to ask questions, or indicate location or possession (see Table 2.1). A more detailed review of this sequence of development follows.

Table 2.1 Levels in children's language development

Levels	Language development
Preverbal	Early vocalizing and non-vocal activity: parents attach meaning to infant actions and sounds that are not yet intentional
Level 1	Preliminary skills • looking together • turn-taking and imitation • appropriate play
Level 2	Preverbal skills • gestures (pointing) • performatives ('oh-oh', 'br'mm br'mm') • protowords (non-conventional or 'made up' words)
Level 3	First words ('dog', 'Mum', 'car')
Level 4	Early sentences ('Daddy car', 'dog gone', 'boy fall down'; 'cat go there')
Level 5	Extending meaning (adding morphemes, such as the English plural 's' as in 'dogs')

Preverbal level: early vocalizing; adults attach meaning to actions and sounds that are not yet intentional

As noted in the previous chapter, the origins of language development can be traced to the infant's earliest experiences. Studies of babies during the very earliest stages of development (e.g. Halliday, 1975; Greenfield and Smith, 1976; Trevarthen, 1979; Kaye, 1982) have shown that the foundations of language are laid when infants start to show an interest in people and in the objects that surround them. They learn to follow a carer's gaze, to see what he or she is looking at. They also learn that when something interesting attracts their attention, the carer will notice their interest and comment on it, or move them closer so that they can touch the object or see it more closely. Infants are very interested in anything that is unusual or different. They like complicated patterns and will look longer at things that are colourful, move, or make interesting noises.

Infants' first apparently 'communicative' acts often take the form of cries and calls, often triggered by physical events such as hunger, cold or colic. They make different sounds when they are tired or in pain, and parents often interpret these sounds to mean that the baby is hungry or wants to be comforted. It is some months before the infant can actually produce sounds intentionally to indicate pleasure, hunger or pain.

From soon after birth, carers begin to attribute meaning to these early sounds: 'the baby's hungry, tired, upset'. These judgements are often based on context, such as 'baby is crying and it is four hours since the last feed so she must be hungry' or past experience as in 'yesterday he cried like this after a feed and finally went to sleep for a long time'. Very young babies also learn to gurgle and coo, and make other interesting sounds for their own entertainment; these noises can often be heard when they are alone, either before or after a nap. Of course, carers cannot know what causes infant behaviour and their interpretations may not be accurate. But over time, as they respond consistently to infants' actions and sounds, the first steps towards social interaction and communication begin.

Level 1: Preliminary skills: looking together, turn-taking and imitation; appropriate play

From about 6 months of age, most infants begin to learn that sounds can be used pragmatically, to make things happen around them. At about this time, they are also acquiring more complex strategies for exploring and interacting with their environment and learning about the objects and people in it. Initially, they learn about objects by putting everything into their mouths, but gradually they learn to drop, give, wave them, bang them together, and so on. Eventually, these strategies become more complex; the spoon is put into the cup, the blanket is piled up on top of the teddy and pillow. Objects can now be picked up, as well as dropped, and small items can be held one in each hand at the same time. Some of these actions are learned by accident; others are learned by watching and participating with others in daily routines like eating, bathing or dressing. At these times, the child and an adult or other children often look together at interesting objects or events such as a new bath toy that pops up out of the water, a book with flaps that can be lifted up. They also take part in games such as 'Boo' or 'Incy, Wincy Spider' that involve the infant and partner in taking turns or in imitations of each other's actions and sounds.

In all of these experiences, babies are learning about the people, objects, events and sounds in their world. They are learning that balls can be dropped or put into a bucket and are sometimes blue and sometimes red; that balls can be rolled back and forth to a partner. They are learning that particular sounds are associated with specific objects or actions or events, such as the 'ring ring' of the telephone and 'oh-oh' when something falls down. They learn that the words that they hear represent or 'stand for' particular referents such as 'Daddy', 'ball', 'phone', 'more', 'gone' and 'fall down' (Hollich, Hirsh-Pasek and Golinkoff, 2000). At the same time, they take the first steps in expressive language by learning that they can use actions and sounds to make things happen. If they cry long and loud enough, someone will come; if they stretch out and point to something interesting, someone will bring it closer or lift them up to see it better; if they call 'more', someone will play the ball game again.

Early games are also very important for language development because they give adults topics that they can talk about when they are with infants; experiences that both have shared. Of course, these games also give the infants something that they can share with the adults who interact with them; 'boo' will remind an older sibling to play the game again and 'open' might remind Daddy to read the book with the pages that unfold wide. Learning to talk involves more than learning about objects; it also involves learning to interact with other people, sharing ideas, remembering past experiences as well as asking for help or information. It also involves learning to express intentions within a social context.

Communication involves interaction with others, so infants need to learn to take turns in activities with others: 'my turn to roll the ball; now it's your turn'. They also need to learn to watch others and imitate what they are doing, since imitation is a powerful tool for acquiring new behaviours. Joining in activities with others is the best way to acquire these skills.

Level 2: Preverbal skills – gestures: pointing; performatives: 'oops'; protowords: non-conventional or 'made up' words

Gestures

Gestures are actions that are made with the intention of communicating meaning and are part of the pragmatic aspect of language. They can involve hands, fingers, face and the whole body and are often accompanied by eye contact and vocalizations. Bates and her associates (Bates, 1976; Bates et al., 1979) demonstrated that children use gestures to express meaning in two ways:

- to *indicate* the existence of something (object, person or event) sometimes referred to as 'deictic gestures
- to *represent* things that are known to exist, as in outstretched arms to 'signify' an aeroplane, or for culturally defined meanings such as waving the hand for 'bye bye'.

Indicative or deictic gestures appear first and are used to either engage the help of another person in order to obtain a desired objective (proto-imperative gestures) or as a strategy for gaining attention (proto-declarative gestures). An example of the first is the child looking towards her mother, stretching out her arm towards a box of felt pencils, fingers opening and shutting to indicate that she wants a pen for drawing on the paper. An example of the second is the child plucking a leaf or a flower, or picking up a stone or a shell and giving it to a carer, as if to say 'Look at this!' or 'Here I am. Look at what I have given you'.

Representational gestures appear later and have the function of both establishing reference to a specific entity and representing a fixed meaning (Iverson and Thal, 1998). The gestures that children use often share a characteristic of the referent, as in the outspread arms of an aeroplane. Hand waving is a socially accepted movement used to indicate farewells. Initially, the meaning intended by the child is quite limited but over time, it is extended, as when the 'plane' gesture is used to indicate a bird or butterfly and the 'bye bye' gesture to indicate 'time to go home' or 'finished'. This is evidence of the tendency for children to extend a known word to refer to similar or related entities. As the child learns to utter intelligible words, gestures and words are used in a complementary way with little overlap between the meanings expressed by each method of communication. Both function to expand the range of meanings that the child is able to communicate.

Gestures appear at about the same time as other forms of representational behaviour. For example, the child who has learned to wave 'bye bye' will also be likely to wave fingers to represent and accompany 'Twinkle Twinkle Little Star'. Performative sounds and single words will begin to be used at about the same time.

Performatives

Performatives, sometimes called *vocables* (Ferguson, 1978) are ritualized sounds, often linked to actions or entities that are associated with a specific sound, such as 'whee' when sliding down a slippery slide, 'br'mm' while pushing a toy car, or 'woof woof' when looking at a picture of a dog. They usually involve a repeated pattern that is easy to remember and sounds that are easy to produce such as 'sh-sh ' and 'er-er' when rocking and 'oh-oh' when something falls down. They are 'event bound' in that they are usually associated with particular events, as in 'chuff chuff' with the model train and 'ping ping ping' with the microwave (Barrett, 1995).

The earliest signs of language appear when an infant begins to combine contact with objects and interactions with adults in one event. For example, Alex has watched entranced as a wind-up car turned circles and has also watched his father wind it up and activate it. Later, he will attract his father's attention to activate the toy by using a consistent gesture such as pointing, or sound such as 'er-er'. The production of performatives is a sign that Alex is gaining some control over the sounds that he is able to make.

Infants gain information about performative sounds when they begin to attend to what is happening around them, not only what can be seen, but also what can be heard. The microwave makes an interesting 'ping', the telephone rings, the washing machine goes 'beep beep'. The dog's bark sounds like 'woof' and the cat makes a 'miaou' noise. Learning about the different events in their lives involves learning about the sounds, sight, touch, taste and smell of these events. When they remember what they have seen and heard, they recall many of these sensory traces.

Gradually, infants begin to use the sounds that they have learned to represent the objects and events that they are associated with. For example, if you push the toy car, you can make a 'br'mm' noise. When you make the 'br'mm' noise and point, Mummy will get the toy car out of the cupboard. If Auntie comes to visit, 'boo' will remind her to play the hiding game and when Daddy comes he will show you his watch if you say 'tick tick'. Most children produce these early sounds in the period before their first words. Initially, the sounds have no meaning; for example, 'boo' and 'boomps-a-daisy'. Eventually, the sounds begin to be used to represent the game or activity with which they are associated. Later, these early sounds will be replaced by proper words, but in the earliest stages of language acquisition they provide a very useful transition into first words.

Protowords

Protowords are word-like vocalizations used intentionally in a consistent context to convey a specific meaning (McCarthy, 1954, cited by Ingram, 1989, pp. 170–1). Halliday (1975) argued that they are created by children from their own vocalizing, as a means of expressing their own meaning. Examples could include the sounds used for a favourite toy or food. These words are not like the words they replace but they have recognizable tone and pitch. They are often used when the child has discovered that words can be used to achieve a purpose, such as to attract attention or obtain a desired object, but has not yet learned to produce the appropriate sounds. Twins sometimes develop quite extensive private communication systems using protowords. However, children need to learn the language of their group so that they can communicate with people outside the family. Eventually, more conventional word forms are acquired, as when 'car' replaces 'br'mm br'mm' or 'bottle' is used instead of a sucking noise or a non-conventional word created by the child.

Some children begin to talk by using word-like vocalizations that are used in place of real words. Everyone in the family eventually learns what is meant when these word-like sounds are used. Protowords are usually just another form of communicative behaviour that precedes first words.

According to Halliday (1975), children use early 'word-like' sounds and later, first words to fulfil a basic set of purposes or functions:

- *instrumental*: 'I want'
- *regulatory*: 'do as I tell you'

- *interactional*: 'me and you'
- *personal*: 'here I am'.

These developments are considered in more detail in Chapter 10.

Level 3: First words: 'dog', 'mum', 'car'

The first words produced by children often seem to be used sporadically, over a period of time, and are only intelligible to a primary carer. These words are usually labels for objects and people, as in 'car', 'Mummy', although a range of other words are also acquired to represent actions 'up', 'see'; locations 'there', 'down', 'in'; modifiers 'hot', 'big', 'there'; and other socially useful meanings such as 'bye', 'no', 'more'.

There is some evidence (e.g. Nelson, 1973; Dore, 1978) that children's initial interests in objects and people are shaped by the major orientations of their primary carers. Some children seem to use more general object labels first, whereas others are more interested in social activities and the regulation of another's behaviour. These differences can frequently also be observed in their carers (Dore, 1978). Observational records show that, whereas children in the first group produce words such as 'dog', 'ball', 'car', those in the second group are more likely to produce words that are useful in social interaction, such as 'hi', 'bye', 'nite-nite', or socially appropriate formulaic expressions such as 'have-a-cup-of-tea?' or 'how-do-you-do?' The latter are often uttered in a continuous stream with the appropriate intonation but the individual words unintelligible.

It is important to remember, here, that while carers are usually very interested in pinpointing when a child actually begins to talk, as in 'I'll give her a canary when she says her first word!', this interest is focused on only one aspect of language use, namely, expressive language skills. Of equal importance is the child's acquisition of receptive language or the skills needed to listen to and comprehend language. Studies of word comprehension in infants and young children (e.g. Benedict, 1979; Bates, Bretherton and Snyder, 1988; Bates, Dale and Thal, 1995) suggest that children begin to understand words well before they are able to use them. Interestingly, the first words that children understand appear to be mainly words associated with actions, such as give, get, no, kiss (Benedict, 1979). On the other hand, as noted above, the first words that they produce are more likely to be general or specific labels for significant people or objects such as 'Daddy', 'Mummy', 'dog', 'cat', 'car', 'ball', 'shoes' (Nelson, 1973).

Level 4: Combining words into sentences: early sentences, 'Daddy car', 'dog gone'

Once children have about 50 words in their spoken vocabulary and understand almost 200 words (Bates, Dale and Thal, 1995), they begin to combine them into simple sentences in a sequence that directly reflects their experience or perception of the world. At first, words are produced separately, as two single words on the same topic, each with a distinct intonation pattern. Later, the words begin to merge into a coherent string. Soon afterwards, children combine them into a single utterance.

Children usually combine words into two-word phrases in predictable ways. The words used represent the semantic categories: agent, action and object. They can also be described in terms of grammatical categories such as noun and verb. The first single words used are mainly general labels that represent a variety of meanings. For example, 'drink' can mean a glass of milk or the act of drinking. Later, action words are acquired such as 'eat', 'go', 'fall-down'. These are then combined in different ways with labels for people and objects, as in 'eat bickie, 'go car', 'Winnie fall-down'. The next step is to add words that modify the object labels, such as 'more bickie', 'my ball' and 'little car'. Other useful words are learned, including words to greet and farewell ('hi', 'bye'), to describe ('wet', 'little', 'yellow'), to show possession ('my', 'mine'), to indicate location ('there', 'that', 'up'). These are then combined with other words to express a specific meaning more clearly. The sentences are formed by following familiar word-combination patterns (Howe, 1993).

Children's first two-word combinations can be described as following a pattern that is comparable to an event script (Nelson, 1986; Shank and Abelson, 1977; see also Chapter 3). The child first learns the main elements of the event, such as getting undressed, getting into the bath and getting out, for 'having a bath'. Later, other components are added, such as whether soap or bubbles are put into the bath, which toys go into the bath and so on. These less critical, more varied parts of the bath script are called 'slot-fillers'. For the child who is learning to talk, key action words such as 'go', 'see' and 'eat' are combined with a variety of labels for objects, people's names and other types of words as in 'daddy go', 'go car', 'see cat', 'Mummy see', 'eat (ba)nana', 'Jamie eat', 'eat more'. Later, as the child's speech becomes more fluent, the listener will begin to hear multi-word utterances that include even longer chains of key words linked with different slot-fillers. These different semantic combinations demonstrate the gradual emergence of rule-bound speech.

After children learn two-word phrases to express a variety of meanings, they begin to combine these to produce sentences of three words or more, such as:

'me want' + 'want drink' = 'me want drink'.
'go car' + 'Mummy car' = 'go Mummy car'

At this stage children can express more detailed information by the use of modifying words for colour, size, possession and so on, as in 'me go big red car', 'want my blue ball'.

Level 5: Extending meaning: using English morphemes, plural 's', present progressive 'ing'

At about the same time as children begin to combine words into sentences, they also begin to acquire morphemes or the small words or parts of words. These are used to add meaning to other words, such as a plural '-s' or '-es', prepositions such as 'in' and 'on' and articles such as 'a' and 'the'. According to Brown (1973), the first to appear is '-ing', followed by 'in', 'on' and the plural 's'. For the child, the addition of a morpheme to a word, as in the addition of '-ing' to make 'eating' or 'sitting' is the equivalent of saying two single words. So examples of 'two-word' combinations produced at this time might include: 'putting', 'washed', 'shoes', 'a cup'.

Once children can combine words into more complex sentences there is often a rapid expansion, both in the size of their vocabulary and in their overall language skills. They are now learning to use language in a variety of ways: to ask and answer questions, to give and get information, to protest and to discover new words. These pragmatic uses of language began much earlier, when the child learned to use sounds, gestures and words to draw the attention of others to objects and events of interest, to obtain desired objects or help, and to protest or attract attention. Dore (1978) and Halliday (1975) have described the different communicative functions of language in greatest detail. These are also discussed in Chapter 10.

Once children are using language in more complex ways, both in terms of pragmatic functions and the range of morphemes observed in their utterances, it can be assumed that they have mastered the most difficult tasks in learning to talk. Further progress will involve expanding the lexicon and learning to use more complex aspects of the grammatical system.

Summary

In this chapter, the levels that children pass through as they learn to talk are described and reference is made to the ways in which adults help in this process. It is important to have some idea of these levels when beginning to help a child who is having language difficulties. For example, how do children move from just looking at interesting things with adults to being able to use words as part of a game or to describe what they are doing? If we can understand what is happening as such developments take place, then we can use this knowledge to help children who are experiencing difficulties to progress in the same way.

In the next two chapters, we shall look more carefully at the way in which adult–child interaction and the context in which it occurs contribute to the development of early language skills.

Chapter 3
Contexts for learning: routine events and play

This chapter is concerned with the contexts in which children acquire language. These include situations in which they learn new skills, but also those where they practise what they have already learned. Many of these contexts involve daily routines at home. They also include other times when children and adults interact, talk, look at a book or play a finger game such as 'Round and Round the Garden' or 'This Little Piggy'. Other important contexts for language involve activities described as 'play'.

Play is particularly important for children who are learning to talk. It provides situations within which real learning can occur, where children have both the time and the opportunity to explore thoroughly new objects and materials, to discover new ideas and test what they have learned in a safe environment that they can control. Play provides opportunities for children to be challenged in their thinking and learn how to solve problems. It is also the best place to learn how to interact successfully with others.

The chapter begins with a review of two research studies that explored the relationship between specific contexts and children's use of language. This is followed by a discussion of the significance of naturally occurring situations, including daily routines, stories, action songs, nursery rhymes and play as contexts for encouraging and practising early language skills. The characteristics of children's play at different levels of language development are described and the role of parents and other carers in children's play is considered.

Contexts for learning to talk

As noted in earlier chapters, children learn to talk by taking part in activities within the natural environment that involve interacting with others who can provide good models of appropriate language. Many of these situations occur daily: while eating breakfast, having a bath, waiting for the bus. Others occur during games and social activities when children interact with adults and other children. Within these contexts partners follow the child's lead, modelling appropriate actions, sounds and words, taking turns with the child to throw a ball, push a car or put another block on the tower. They are also responsive to the child's attempts to communicate.

Studies of children's language development have demonstrated an association between specific natural contexts and language use. For example, Wells (1985) in a longitudinal study of Bristol families, tape-recorded samples of children's language in their homes over a three-year period, beginning when the children were aged around 15 months (younger group) and 39 months (older group). In exploring the relationship between language use and context, Wells showed that the most speech occurred in domestic 'non-play' situations where the child was simply an observer and not directly involved in any activity. Over 20 per cent of all the speech recorded in this study occurred in such contexts. A relatively high percentages of speech also occurred when the child was playing alone (self-talk) or with other children, or while simply 'talking' with an adult (being engaged in a conversation).

Among the daily routines that children experienced, speech occurred most often during eating, dressing and toileting. From around 42 months, children began to talk more when they were 'helping' an adult. Interestingly, the percentage of speech associated with looking at books and reading decreased over the time period observed. Wells comments that this activity was, at first, used by parents to teach children vocabulary. It gradually declined as the children's language skills began to develop more rapidly.

Sylva, Roy and Painter (1980) also identified specific contexts associated with high and low language use. As in Wells' study, observations were made of children (aged 3–5 years), but in this case, the children were attending nursery schools, nursery classes and playgroups in the Oxford area. These data showed that child–adult exchanges occurred most often when the children were engaged in tasks associated with early attempts at reading, writing and counting and, to a lesser extent, with structured materials such as puzzles, pegboards and posting boxes. The highest rate of child–child language occurred during informal games where children held hands and giggled, hid in corners and took part in activities described as 'rough and tumble'. The children were most likely to be silent when engaged in adult-directed activities where the aim was to improve skills such as cutting, tracing, pasting and colouring in, and during activities that involved manipulation of materials such as sewing, sorting or playing with dough or water.

The results of the studies by Wells and Sylva et al. confirm that language interaction tends to occur more often in some contexts than in others. At home, most language occurs at times when children are interested, but not always directly involved, in some ongoing domestic activity, or when they converse with an adult about topics of interest. Mealtimes also provide opportunities for conversation. In an early childhood setting, the most child–adult exchanges occur when children are not physically involved in an activity, or when they are involved with tasks that require relatively high levels of concentration. Such tasks include pre-reading and mathematics, and structured materials involving fine motor skills and eye–hand coordination such as puzzles and pegboards.

Not unexpectedly, children talk less with adults when involved in gross motor activities such as running, climbing, chasing and jostling. They are also less talkative during tasks that require very high concentration and fine motor skills, such as playing with plastic building bricks (Lego). Activities that involve coordination of fine movements and senses such as sand, dough and water, or sorting and arranging objects are less conducive to language. Children are most likely to talk with other children during informal games.

Daily routines and familiar situations

In earlier chapters we talked about the way in which children learn about objects and people. For example, they learn about balls by playing with balls and they learn to recognize the characteristics that distinguish Mummy, Daddy or a regular carer from other people by their look, sound, smell, touch and so on. Children also learn about their daily life by recognizing the pattern of recurring events. They learn what happens first and what happens next, what they have to do and what others do. They are often more interested in sorting out these sequences ('now I have breakfast, then I go to playgroup') than in the more unusual and exciting things that engage the interest of adults, such as the birth of a sibling or a forthcoming holiday. Nelson (1989) gives a fascinating account of the topics covered by a 2-year-old child during pre-sleep monologues. Children acquire what has been called 'event knowledge' as they learn about the different activities that they take part in each day, such as having a bath, going to bed, visiting the doctor or going to the shops (e.g. Nelson and Gruendel, 1979). All of these events involve a fairly predictable sequence of actions, as well as having a predictable set of words to accompany the actions. These words can be used as goals in a language programme for a child who needs help in early communication.

The sequence of actions and words that recur within daily routines and familiar events are sometimes referred to as forming a 'script' of the routine or event. For example, a possible script for having a bath is given in Table 3.1. Obviously, not every bath will follow the set of actions and words outlined here. Each family will have its own procedure and that sequence will be repeated every time the child is bathed. The main events of taking off clothes, filling the tub, washing, getting out, drying, dressing and emptying the bath will be shared by many children. The language that accompanies the actions will also be fairly similar for a particular child and carer and can be targeted during activities designed to encourage the acquisition of new language skills. For example, the child at the performative level can be encouraged to say 'sh-sh-sh' as the tap is turned on; the child at the single-word level can practise saying 'in', 'finished', 'out' and so on.

Table 3.1 A script for having a bath

Actions	Language
Put in plug and turn water on	'plug in', 'water on/off', 'sh-sh-sh'
Take clothes off	'shirt off', 'pants off'
Get in bath	'in'
Wash, play with bath toys	'wash face/arms/legs', 'boat', 'woosh', 'duck', 'quack quack'
Get out	'finished', 'out'
Dry face/body/arms/legs	'pat pat', 'rub rub'
Empty bath	'plug out', 'gurgle gurgle', 'water gone'

Other recurring events that could provide useful opportunities to encourage and practise new language skills include:

• waking up and getting dressed
• mealtimes
• visits to aunts, uncles, grandparents
• arriving and leaving crèche, playgroup, preschool
• going shopping
• going for a walk
• going to church
• having a picnic
• birthdays
• eating at McDonald's
• getting ready for bed
• saying goodnight.

You can think of other similar activities that children and their carers take part in together, and of the sequence of actions and words that the child is learning to associate with these events. These scripts can be used during imaginary play involving replication of daily routines. They will also be useful when you begin to select language goals, and plan activities to learn and practise new language skills.

Stories, action songs and nursery rhymes

Familiar stories, read or told, songs and nursery rhymes, particularly those that accompany physical movements such as bouncing on the knees or finger play, provide another context for language acquisition. When such experiences are repeated many times, children become familiar with the structure and content of stories and songs that they hear.

As adults, we generally read a newspaper article or a book only once, unless it has particular significance or is a favourite. However, children enjoy repetition of favourite stories, nursery rhymes, and songs. They learn the words, rhymes and rhythms, and can predict the relevant script or schema for the story (Mandler and Johnson, 1977), who the actors are and what will happen first, next and last. As in the example of script-learning arising from participation in recurring daily routines, so, too, repetition of favourite stories, songs and rhymes gives children opportunities to remember predictable sequences of actions and associated words and sound patterns. These experiences are highly motivational. They also provide children with valuable opportunities to practise their language in a safe and predictable environment.

If the story includes the repetition of specific words, as in *The Three Bears* ('Who's been eating my porridge?'), the children do not even have to find appropriate language, but can just say the words used in the story. If they sing a familiar song such as 'Twinkle, Twinkle Little Star' or 'Happy Birthday to You', a listener will quickly recognize the tune, if not the words, and respond appropriately. These experiences can be a useful place to begin to encourage talking. Ideas for using stories, songs and nursery rhymes for encouraging and practising early language-related skills are included in Chapter 6.

Children's play

To many adults, 'play' is thought of as something that we do when we are free to decide how to spend our time. Play is something that is fun, where we can follow our own interests. There are no fixed goals and, as a result, little possibility of frustration or failure (Sylva, Bruner and Genova, 1976; Elkind, 1990; Butterfield, 1994). In contrast, 'work' is usually associated with tasks that have a specific goal and, with this, the potential for frustration and failure if the goal is not achieved. There is usually little flexibility about the way the task is carried out and participation is not always voluntary. The distinction between children's 'play' and their 'work' is worth keeping in mind when considering suggestions for engaging children in 'play' activities as a means of encouraging and practising new skills and behaviours. Children may be more willing to join in the game if they know it will be fun.

When children are left to amuse themselves, to do what they like with their time, we usually describe their activity as 'play', but can all of the things that children do at these times be described in this way? Is it also possible to distinguish between different types of play in children's activity? Can you tell when children are 'playing' and when they are not? What is the function of play? Which are the more effective play contexts for language learning?

According to Piaget (1962), play provides children with a means to assimilate or incorporate new information into existing knowledge. Montessori (1967) described play as children's 'work'. Such descriptions are supported by evidence that children attend more carefully to unfamiliar rather than familiar experiences and are more likely to express emotion following new or unexpected play activities. So it is possible to distinguish between play as intrinsically motivating engagement in familiar activities and as a means of acquiring new knowledge and interpreting new experiences (Lifter and Bloom, 1998). Studies of 3–4-year-olds in preschools (e.g. Hutt et al., 1989) have shown that differences can be identified in the various activities that the children engage in during periods that we might call 'play'. Some activities are chosen because they are fun. Their main purpose is self-amusement (Hutt et al., 1989, p. 12). Children involved in such activities are relaxed and happy; their behaviour is unpredictable and sometimes highly creative or unusual. When these activities cease to be fun, the children simply stop doing them. Examples of such games include playing with trains and model cars, tea parties, doll's corner, dressing-up and imaginative games where children assume different roles in an interaction.

Other types of play activity that children become involved in are mainly concerned with acquiring information. Such games require very high levels of concentration, as, for example, during exploration of unfamiliar materials, acquisition of new skills and problem-solving. During this type of play, children's attention is highly focused and their actions are very predictable. Examples of such activities include finding out how to start a new mechanical toy, making something like a rocket out of boxes, learning new skills such as riding a tricycle or skipping, and solving problems as in finishing a puzzle or threading beads to match a pattern.

Sometimes children who have been left to play do not seem to be doing anything. They wander about indecisively or flit from one activity to another, not really being involved in anything. These children may not yet have decided what to do with their playtime, but they may also not know how to play or may be simply 'played out' (Linn, Goodman and Lender, 2000). Most children learn how to play by watching other children or adults and imitating what they are doing.

Interestingly, studies of children's play often report relatively high percentages of time spent by children in 'looking' and 'watching'. For example, Hutt et al. (1989, p. 72) reported that over 20 per cent of the time spent by the children they observed in nursery schools, nursery classes, playgroups and day nurseries was engaged in this type of activity. Some of these children may not previously have had opportunities to watch other children playing. They will become more active when they feel confident enough to join in. However, some children lack the skills needed to learn spontaneously from simple observation. Such children need access to stimulating environments, and in some cases, assistance or 'scaffolding', as suggested by Vygotsky (Bodrova and Leong, 1996) to ensure that they benefit from periods of 'watching and looking'. The term 'scaffolding' is used to describe the behaviour of a responsive adult when interacting with a young child. The adult's aim is to involve the child in dialogue and to provide a context or meaning for the child's gestures and early utterances. One of the adult's tasks is to adjust the interchange to ensure the participation of an immature partner. Scaffolding assists the child to acquire more advanced skills.

Of course, it is not always possible to tell why children are doing something or whether they are really enjoying what they are doing. Sometimes the children themselves are not sure; the different kinds of games are mixed up together. Nevertheless, it is often possible to distinguish between the different types of play in children's games. In general, 'play' that takes the form of self-amusement has the following characteristics; it is:

- *fun*: children stop playing when the game is no longer enjoyable
- *voluntary*: children play because they want to, not because they have to
- *flexible*: goals can change: what children do is the most important part of the game
- *has no failure*: achieving a goal is not important; you can 'lose', as in chasing or catching games, but you cannot 'fail' during play. (Sylva, Bruner and Genova, 1976, p. 244–5).

When children's activities do not conform to these four qualities (when they are not enjoyable, voluntary, flexible and without failure) then they are probably more like 'work' for the children involved and will require greater cognitive, social and emotional effort. So if you sit down to play with a child and find that you are directing the game, setting the rules and insisting that the child 'finishes' what she is doing, there is a risk that the activity will not seem like fun. When introducing a new activity, you need to ensure that it is enjoyable to the child. You can encourage participation, but do not insist if the child is not interested.

Why is play so useful for helping children to learn to talk? In the early stages of learning to talk, children need to have some control over the situations that they are in. They need to learn that they can use their own actions or sounds intentionally to make things happen. They have to understand that we use particular sounds and gestures to represent specific objects, people and events. They also have to learn to produce the sounds and gestures themselves, in order to have the means to interact with others; for example, to say 'boo' and pull the cloth off your face, instead of always waiting for an adult to pull the cloth and say the word. This learning can occur during daily routines when you and the child share an enjoyable activity. In other words, when early communication skills are being encouraged, activities need to provide a context that encourages children to communicate because they want to and are involved in a shared activity with a partner.

Later, when you begin to help children who can already talk to improve specific aspects of their language, the activities you chose for practising new skills can be more formal and 'work-like'. There can now be an expectation that the child will make an effort to stay and finish the task, in spite of the fact that it may be difficult and not much fun.

Learning to play

In Chapter 2, we described some of the changes that take place as children learn to talk; progressing from the preverbal skills of taking turns, imitation and so on, to more complex verbal skills such as asking and answering questions. In the same way, children's development in learning to play can be seen in terms of their progression through a series of levels.

Currently, much of our understanding about the development of children's play skills is based on the work of Jean Piaget (1962), who observed his own children very carefully and from the knowledge gained, developed a theory about how children learn. Piaget's ideas are useful in drawing attention to the ways in which young children explore and learn about the objects that they encounter around them. Most children progress through this level of learning relatively quickly, but those whose development is slow in some areas, including language, are also sometimes slow in developing these exploratory play skills. Such children may need help to move on to more advanced play and language levels.

In the following discussion, the characteristics of children's play skills at different developmental levels are described. The relationship between these levels of play and the levels of language development outlined in Chapter 2, Table 2.1, is set out in Table 3.2.

Levels of play

Exploring objects or simple actions with one object

Initially, infants seem to learn about objects in their immediate environment by looking very intently and by exploring them using their mouths. As skills in grasping and holding skills improve they will wave objects in front of their eyes, drop them or, as they learn to release things at will, give them to you. At this stage, infants' ability to learn about objects is limited by their physical skills in grasping, holding and releasing.

Combining objects

Gradually, manipulative skills improve and infants begin to use more complex strategies to explore the things that they encounter. They learn to hold two objects at the same time and then combine them in some way.

Table 3.2: Levels of children's language development and play

Level	Language development			Play
Preverbal	Early vocalizing and non-vocal activity: parents attach meaning to infant actions and sounds that are not yet intentional			
Level 1	Preliminary skills			Exploring objects
	Looking together	Turn-taking imitation	Appropriate play	Combining objects Using objects in play
Level 2	Pre-verbal skills • gestures (pointing) • performatives ('oh-oh', 'br'mm br'mm') • protowords (non-conventional or 'made up' words			Functional use of objects Simple pretending using real objects
Level 3	First words ('dog', 'Mum', 'car')			Simple pretending using substitute or imaginary objects
Level 4	Early sentences ('Daddy car', 'dog gone', 'boy fall down', 'cat go there')			Imaginary play
Level 5	Extending meaning (adding English morphemes, such as plural 's' as in 'dogs')			

For example, they will put the spoon into the cup, bang two objects together or put one object on top of another, as when a blanket is piled on a pillow or one block is carefully placed on top of another. Now, you can help them learn to 'put in', 'pull out', 'put on' and so on. Gradually, the children begin to explore the things around them, seeking out new objects and new ways of using material already encountered. The traditional activity of exploring the kitchen cupboard is a good example of appropriate play at this level. Playing with water and sand is also exciting as the children learn, among other things, what can and cannot go into the mouth.

Functional use of objects

By this level, infants have acquired some knowledge of the ways in which familiar objects are used. If you give them a cup they will attempt to drink from it, and they will use a hairbrush to brush their own or your hair. They have usually learned that a book is opened and the pages turned, and know that the sight of their bottle and blanket means that it is time to go to bed. If you want to know something about the language skills of children at this level of development, give them a toy telephone. Most children will immediately lift the receiver and begin to babble. They have watched adults use a telephone and will imitate what they have seen.

Once children have reached this level they need a variety of materials such as tea-sets, toy cars and farm animals that can be used in simple lifelike games that can lead into creative or pretend play.

Simple pretending: real objects

Once children have begun to associate specific play routines with partic-ular objects, they are ready to begin to take part in games that involve simple pretending. Examples include 'drinking' from an empty cup, 'eat-ing' the cakes in the picture book and even 'feeding' teddy and 'putting him to sleep', wrapped up in a blanket. At this stage, the children should be using performative sounds in their games, such as pretend drinking and eating noises to accompany their actions.

Simple pretending: imaginary objects

Early games involving appropriate use of real objects are gradually replaced by games using substitute or imaginary ones. Children are now able to use small pebbles to represent the cakes needed for tea and will happily put teddy to sleep in a box. Single words begin to be used during these games.

Imaginary play

Children move into the creative-symbolic level by extending their games with teddy, the tea-set, the farm animals, the garage, the train set and other culturally appropriate objects and activities. Functional play becomes imaginative as children pretend to have a tea party with a fairy, set up the train so that people can go for a trip to the moon, make a box into a space rocket or build a pirate ship and set sail to find treasure. At this level, children should be combining words into sentences and taking part in conversations.

Parents and carers as managers

Many parents and other carers spend much of their time directing chil-dren, telling them what to do, or how and when to do it. This tendency to 'manage' is a particular problem when children are developing slowly or are having problems in some area of learning. In this situation, it can be very difficult for carers to stop managing and leave the children to choose what they want to do for themselves. To compound this problem, children who are developing slowly often have not developed the skills needed to play independently; to explore and learn about objects and begin to enjoy using them in different 'fun' ways.

One of the main things that parents and other carers need to do if they are to help children begin to learn to talk is to recognize that they will need to spend time interacting with their children. This will include the opportunities that arise naturally, during daily routines such as washing up, washing the car, gardening and going for a walk. It may also involve special times in the day. The best conditions for children to begin to explore and learn about new objects, and then use their new knowledge in creative ways, is when they are in familiar situations that they can control, where they feel safe and in the company of children and adults whom they know well. The best place to learn to talk, for most children, is in a familiar context, either home or another setting, and during activities with parents or carers who are closely involved in their daily life.

Summary

Experience working with children who are having problems in the early stages of learning to talk has demonstrated the importance of natural environments as contexts for language acquisition. In particular, language is acquired through the child's participation in daily routines and recurring events, such as mealtimes, saying 'goodnight' and going to bed. Other important contexts include the stories, finger plays, nursery rhymes and songs that carers share with children. Finally, children's play provides opportunities for interaction with others, taking turns to roll a ball, knock down a block tower or pour a cup of tea. Parents, teachers and others can learn to use such routine and play situations to help children begin to communicate more effectively. In the next chapter, the way that adults talk to children during these encounters will be explored in terms of its contribution to children's acquisition of language.

Overall, these results suggest that, at home, children talk most when they are essentially spectators in domestic or other ongoing activities. Speech also occurs when a child and adult sit close together and talk. These are the contexts where familiar stories, songs and rhymes are told. Play situations, where children interact with other children, or verbalize aloud about what they are doing, are also important contexts for acquiring and using new language skills. The next chapter examines the daily routines and familiar situations where children spend extended periods of time as appropriate contexts for learning to talk.

Chapter 4
Talking with children

Communication is, by definition, interactive. Children cannot learn language alone. They are dependent on parents or other carers to help them accomplish this most complicated but necessary task. The transactional model of early language acquisition (Sameroff and Chandler, 1975; McLean and Snyder-McLean, 1978) emphasizes the importance of *contingent reciprocal interaction* between infants and their carers in the acquisition of communication skills. Cognitive, social and linguistic changes within the child also contribute to this process. But the transactional model stresses, above all, that children will not learn to talk unless they have a reason to communicate and someone meaningful with whom to interact. Evidence from studies of children placed in long-term residential care at an early age supports this view (Tizard and Hodges, 1978; Bochner, 1986). This chapter is concerned with the role of parents and others in the process of language acquisition. Information is given about children's interest in people and the sounds of speech, the way adults interact with children acquiring early language skills and the strategies that can be used to encourage effective communication.

Children's interest in people

Research into the earliest interactions between infants and their carers suggests that the origins of communicative behaviour can be traced, in part, to infants' visual and auditory abilities. Although infants are born with their eyes wide open, it used to be assumed that they could not see (Lamb and Campos, 1982). However, it is now known that although their visual capacities are extremely limited when compared with adult vision, infants have an active interest in visual stimulation. Visual development is rapid, approaching adult levels by 3 or 4 months of age (Simion and Butterworth, 1998; Slater, 2000).

Studies of eye movements and fixations in infants show that, from birth, they look longer and more often at moving, three-dimensional, high-contrast and curved stimuli, rather than at stimuli that are stationary, two-dimensional, low-contrast or straight. This means that, from an early age, they prefer to look at faces or face-like patterns. Moreover, they prefer to look at some faces rather than others. For example, even 2-day-old infants look longer at their mother's face than at the face of a strange woman who has been matched with their mother in terms of the general brightness of the face and hair colour. The same effect is found when the faces are in photographs or videos (Bushnell, Sai and Mullin, 1989; Walton, Bower and Bower, 1992). Some time between 4 and 7 months they begin to distinguish between a happy and a sad face on the same model (Nelson, 1987) and between 7 and 10 months they are able to distinguish between positive and negative expressions on different people (Ludemann, 1991).

There is also evidence that from an early age, infant development is influenced by contingency (an action that is conditional on a preceding action), reciprocity (mutual giving and receiving) and communication in their carers. For example, in situations where stimulation is non-contingent (an action that is not conditional on a preceding action), infants' motivation to interact with others is reduced and their ability to recognize adult intentions impaired (Muir and Hains, 1999). They will smile at a person who is interacting with them but not at a hand puppet with moving features and synthesized tone that can be activated contingently (Legerstee, 1992; Ellsworth, Muir and Hains, 1993). At this stage, adult contingent responses can take the form of imitation of the infant's actions, facial expression, or sounds. Reciprocity can take the form of complementary actions during play, vocal turn-taking and vocal acknowledgement as in 'uh huh' or 'm'mm' (Yoder et al., 1998). Following the child's lead is also important in that it results in joint attention by infant and carer to objects or events that interest the child. This shared experience provides one of the essential bases for later acquisition of language. These different carer responses contribute to development of communication skills by encouraging a sense of self in infants, assisting them to learn that their actions have an effect on the world.

Infant familiarity with a carer is important at this early level of development, with visual attention reduced and almost no smiling during interaction with an unfamiliar person. In part, this reduction in attention and affect may be associated with infants' need for a sense of security and attachment, as a base from which to explore the world (Ainsworth et al., 1978; Bowlby, 1982; Thompson, 1998). Eye contact is also important in infants' growing understanding of carer behaviour. By 3 months of age, eye contact from a carer is interpreted by the infant as an indicator of interactive intent by the carer. If the carer looks away, infants will follow their eye movements for information about where to look (Muir and Hains, 1999).

Interest in speech sounds

There is some evidence that infants discriminate speech sounds in terms of rhythm, intonation, pitch and stress (prosodic features) (Cooper and Aslin,

1990). They also attend to rhythm in music (Trehub and Thorpe, 1989). They seem to distinguish syllables in speech sounds, focusing on those parts of a word that are stressed rather than unstressed, discriminating a phrase like 'guitar is' as 'taris' (Newsome and Jusczyk, 1995). Vowel sounds carry most of the information discerned by infants. Apparently, they are able to distinguish details of the duration, pitch and amplitude of vowel sounds. They perceive a string of words as comprising a sequence of vowel sounds with associated rhythm and intonation patterns (Bertoncini, 1998).

Infants' ability to discriminate prosodic elements of speech is reflected in their preference for specific types of sounds. For example, when listening to musical sounds, they prefer high rather than low notes and a range of musical notes rather than a single sound (Eisenberg, 1976). This has important implications for their response to adult speech directed towards them; when adults talk to babies, their speech tends to have a higher and more varied pitch than at other times. From soon after birth, infants demonstrate a preference for this type of speech rather than for the language that occurs between adults (Cooper and Aslin, 1990).

The sound pattern of adult speech to children provides melodic clues about the intention of the speaker (Stern, Spieker and MacKain, 1982; Papousek, Papousek and Haekel, 1987). For example, attempts to gain infant attention are associated with a rising intonation, falling tones to sooth or direct attention, and a rising and falling pattern to maintain attention or reward behaviour. These patterns have been demonstrated across different linguistic groups including English, Mandarin and German (Messer, 1994).

Social interaction

One of the critical functions of mother–infant interaction, particularly in the first 12 months of life, is the opportunity it provides for infants to learn the procedures that provide a framework for later conversation. Through these social experiences, infants learn the rhythms of interaction: the cycles of on-off vocalizing, pausing, looking and looking away. This rhythm may not be strictly regular, but it does have a recurring pattern that is an essential component of communication. It provides infants with opportunities to begin to predict and anticipate the behaviour of another person. This process has been described as involving 'reciprocal interaction' and 'rhythmic coordination' (Jaffe et al., 2001, p. 2).

Motherese

It has long been noticed that adults modify the language they use when interacting with young children (see Snow, 1994). The term 'motherese' ('adultese' or 'parentese', Messer, 1994; Owens, 1996) has been used to describe such speech. Even children as young as 4 years of age modify their speech when interacting with younger, more immature siblings.

Such speech is slower, clearer, more fluent, with shorter, simpler utter-ances, fewer false starts and hesitations, more exaggerated intonation, higher pitch and a greater than usual use of rising tones. Words, phrases and whole utterances are frequently repeated, as a whole or in part, and topics tend to be restricted to present activities, objects and events (Snow, 1994). These strategies are used both to help infants recognize the intent of the speaker and to assist them to begin to differentiate the words that are used. Stress is placed on words that are important semat-ically (usually labels for objects) and such words are often placed at the end of a sentence, thus heightening the likelihood that they will be noticed and remembered by the infant. Studies of mothers reading to their 14-month-old infants demonstrate this pattern of use (Fernald and Mazzie, 1991). Some of the characteristics of motherese are listed in Table 4.1.

Table 4.1 Characteristics of motherese compared with adult-to-adult speech

Paralinguistic	Slower speech with longer pauses between utterances and after content words
	Higher overall pitch; greater pitch range
	Exaggerated intonation and stress
	More varied loudness pattern
	Fewer dysfluencies (one dysfluency per 1000 words versus 4.5 per 1000 for adult–adult)
	Fewer words per minute
Lexical	More restricted vocabulary
	Three times as much paraphrasing
	More concrete reference to here and now
Semantic	More limited range of semantic functions
	More contextual support
Syntactic	Fewer broken or run-on sentences
	Shorter, less complex sentences (approximately 50% are single words or short declaratives)
	More well-formed and intelligible sentences
	Fewer complex sentences
	More imperatives and questions (approximately 60% of utter-ances)
Conversational	Fewer utterances per conversation
	More repetitions (approximately 16% of utterances are repeated within three turns)

Source: Owens (1996), p.219.

Questions that arise from research findings about motherese concern the purpose served by the modifications and adjustments made by adults when they communicate with young children who are acquiring language. Are such modifications essential features of language-learning environ-ments or is it possible for young children to acquire language without them? Do children make use of the language they hear in the same way at different stages in their development as language users? Is adult input the same for children who learn language easily as for those who experience difficulty? Studies designed to clarify these issues have been conducted with mothers of children who are developing normally and mothers whose children are delayed in the area of language. Examples of such research include Mahoney and Robenalt (1986), Mahoney (1988), Tannock (1988) and Andersen, Dunlea and Kekelis (1993).

One way of thinking about the purpose of the adjustments made by adults when they talk to children is in terms of the *function* of such speech. Possible functions for these adjustments identified by Richards and Gallaway (1994, pp. 263–4) include:

- *managing attention* or engaging the child's attention to relevant aspects of the situation
- *promoting positive affect* or feelings of togetherness and warmth
- *improving intelligibility* by modifying intonation and the pace of adult speech to help the child identify single words and sentences
- *giving feedback* about the acceptability of the child's utterances
- *modelling correct utterances* by giving examples of correct speech and appropriate conversational behaviour
- *encouraging participation in conversations* by using scaffolding techniques such as checking on intended meaning and encouraging responses
- *teaching social routines* such as 'hi' and 'bye bye'.

The conversational style of mothers caring for children with intellectual disabilities has been described as taking one of three different forms (Mahoney, 1988). 'Attenders' employ frequent behavioural prompts, directing attention, elaborating their own topic and using grammatical form. 'Responders' use one-word utterances, smiles and laughs, exaggerated facial expression and more exclamations. 'Ignorers' are unresponsive and lack sensitivity to the child's communicative attempts. The communicative style of both 'attenders' and 'ignorers', in particular, may not appear to be the most appropriate for facilitating language skills of these children. However, some aspects of these styles may help to sustain the attention and engagement of children who might otherwise not attend to or participate in relevant activities (Conti-Ramsden, 1994; Messer, 1994).

Studies reported on the outcomes of attempts to modify parents' interactional styles as a means of increasing their children's language skills (Kaiser, 1993; Wetherby, Warren and Reichle, 1998) have provided only tentative guidelines for parents and other carers to follow in their interactions with children who are experiencing problems in learning to talk. However, much has been learned about the ways in which children learn language, the type of social interactions that they engage in, the contribution of their interactive partners, the settings where these exchanges occur and the changes that can be observed as language competence progresses. Even in the absence of appropriate input from adult carers, most children learn to communicate at least adequately for their everyday needs. For children who lack effective input from adults, alternative routes for language acquisition include the routines and associated scripts which structure children's daily lives. This issue is discussed in Chapter 3.

Overall, it is evident that children need many different sources of information in their struggle to learn the meaning and use of words

> much as a baker needs multiple ingredients to make a cake. And as in the culinary arts, the end result is more than any one of the ingredient parts. (Hollich, Hirsh-Pasek and Golinkoff 2000, p. 114).

So although we cannot offer a 'recipe' for language learning, there are many suggestions that can be made to help mothers and other carers facilitate the process of language acquisition through interaction with children.

Encouraging language

Communication begins in infancy, long before a child is able to produce his or her first words. This stage is crucial for later language development because it is the period when all the prerequisite skills are established. Carers are often unaware of the importance of this period. This is the time when mothers interpret infants' signals as if they are meaningful, such as while changing or soothing a crying child. As early patterns of feeding, sleeping and handling are established, carers learn to interpret and respond to infant behaviour, and through this reciprocity infants learn that they can cause things to happen. This is the beginning of joint attention. During this period responsive parents and other carers 'teach' the child that attempts to communicate will be rewarded. This helps to consolidate the child's motivation to want to communicate.

As children's repertoire of actions and sounds increases, responsive adults join in their 'game'. Early sounds are imitated back to the child, introducing the earliest form of turn-taking. Mother will put out her tongue, shake her head and imitate the child's movements and sounds. Again, this involves an interactive sequence that encourages communication. When the child looks at something or points, the adult follows the child's gaze, passing the toy car or touching the mobile to set it moving as if in response to a request to do so. Soon the child makes the gesture or sound with intent, and the interaction becomes truly communicative. When the child raises her arms to be lifted from the cot and the carer says 'up', it is not long before she learns to signal that she wants to be lifted out using the sound 'up' as arms are lifted to say 'take me out of here!'

These early 'games', in the context of the baby and carer's shared interactions in everyday routines, are the basis for all later language learning. The carer is responsive to the child's needs, and to early communicative attempts. As competence increases, gestures turn into sounds, and babbling sounds become more specific. Gradually, the carer extends what is expected of the child, waiting for the sound to go with the gesture before lifting her from the cot. As noted in Chapter 2, this process is sometimes described as 'scaffolding' and helps the child move to a higher level of language use (Vygotsky, 1978).

Responsiveness

The most important factor in facilitating language acquisition is the responsiveness of the carer to the child. This is critical during infancy and continues to be very important at all stages of the child's development. Responsivity has been defined as the rate at which carers respond to a child's gestures, vocalizations or other communicative acts (Yoder and Warren, 2001). A carer's response occurs immediately after the child's communicative act and either complies with it, maps it linguistically, seeks clarification or imitates some component of the child's behaviour (Yoder and Warren, 2001, p. 229). The responsivity of carers engaged in interactive exchanges with a child helps to make the communicative intentions of their partner more 'transparent' to the child (Bruner, 1975; Tomasello, 2001). Where interaction occurs in a non-familiar setting, rather than as part of a routine activity, the carer's input to the conversation provides the infant with information about significant aspects of the situation; the activity that the child is interested in, and any specific meanings that need to be recognized. This helps the child begin to represent aspects of the experience semantically and in turn, contributes to cognitive representation of new concepts, leading eventually to words. There is some evidence that such responsiveness is particularly important in the period before about 18 months. At about this time, infant attention begins to shift to a focus on the semantic rather than the pragmatic content of adult communication, leading to an increase in the size of the lexicon (Hoff and Naigles, 2002).

The 'responsiveness' hypothesis states that the purpose of adult speech is to involve the child in a conversational framework which allows for the child's immature skills. As a result, the child takes part in meaningful interaction with another person and, through this experience, gradually learns the features of the conversational exchange which are appropriate to his or her level of growth. Until these skills are acquired, the adult partner sustains the conversation, maintaining the interaction, allowing time for the child to respond as the topic is negotiated. The longer the topic is maintained, the more opportunities the child has for taking turns. Responding appropriately in terms of the child's topic, mood and pace will encourage further conversation. If new topics are constantly being introduced this opportunity is reduced, and the child has fewer opportunities for feedback. Children play an active role in their language learning, and they need to be assisted and encouraged.

Conversation skills

The complexity of the task of acquiring adequate conversational skills begins in earliest infancy, when the carer infers intent to the baby's pre-intentional sounds and actions. During the first months after birth, infants' interactive skills primarily involve gaze, facial expression and vocalization. Carers provide a 'frame' (Messer, 1994) for these behaviours, varying their facial expression, vocalizations and actions to maintain infant attention and participation in sustained social interaction. Adults also structure these situations by taking both roles in the interaction until the point where infants can take their own turn. This means that, from an early age, children are absorbed into socially interactive encounters that lead to social relationships and a shared view of the world. These experiences provide a solid basis for subsequent acquisition of language skills.

The skills involved in taking part in a conversation are quite complex. Searle (1969) argued that language should be seen as a 'performative' or an action. According to this view, to communicate is, in fact, to act in some way. Examples of Searle's view of 'language as action' can be seen in utterances such as 'I do' in marriage and 'I name' in a christening ceremony. In both instances, the words used represent the action, as in 'to pledge' and 'to label'. According to this view, sounds described as 'speech' have meaning for the speaker and, at the same time, mean something to a listener. For an utterance to have meaning, certain conditions have to be satisfied (Searle, 1969, p. 48):

- the speaker must intend (or mean) what is said
- the speaker chooses words that are conventionally accepted by his speech community
- the listener knows these speech conventions and recognizes the meaning of the words heard
- the listener recognizes (believes) the speaker's intention in using these words
- the speaker recognizes that the listener hears the words, knows their meaning and understands his intention in uttering them
- the listener knows that the speaker recognizes that he has heard that meaning.

This sequence highlights the complexity of participating in a conversation. Not only must the infant grasp at least some elements of this sequence, but must also, having heard the speech sounds uttered by a conversational partner, understand the meaning of the message and:

- think about how to respond
- select the right gesture, sounds or words to reply
- take turns at the appropriate moment
- check to see if the message has been understood.

The whole process is repeated again and again, with increasing competence acquired by the child in selecting the correct gestures, sounds, words or grammatical constructions to convey the intended meaning. The child must also learn when to wait and listen and when to speak and take a turn, how to initiate and obtain the attention of the language partner to share the meanings that are becoming an increasingly important part of social interaction. These skills are an important component of the pragmatic aspect of language or the reasons why language is used.

Triadic conversations

Although many of the conversations that infants engage in involve interaction with a single conversational partner, children may also participate in conversational exchanges that involve a third person – often an older child, often a sibling. These situations are relatively common in the experience of later-born children in a family and those who spend time in daycare and similar settings. Both positive and negative outcomes are associated with these 'triadic' situations. One negative outcome arises from changes in adult speech addressed to the infant, as opposed to speech addressed to the other child or both children. For example, the amount of speech directed to the infant is both greatly reduced in quantity and much less responsive, with greater frequency of directive and controlling utterances (Barton and Tomasello, 1991). The number of infant vocalizations is also reduced (Woollett, 1986). These effects have also been observed in studies of twins interacting with their mothers (Tomasello, Mannle and Kruger, 1986) as well as in situations involving an infant and an older sibling. Beneficial effects can also be seen in triadic interaction. The conversations are much longer than in adult–infant exchanges, and there is also an increase in infant turns during the exchange. Once the infants have acquired some verbal skills, they begin to contribute topic-related comments and responses to these three-way exchanges.

Overall, conversations involving a primary carer, an infant and a sibling or other child provide opportunities for the infant to participate in longer conversations than previously (Barton and Tomasello, 1994). This effect probably results, in part, from the more advanced language skills of the other child who is able to take a more active role in the exchange, modelling more complex vocabulary and language structures. These experiences enhance the infant's skills in joining in conversations that involve more than one speaker, an invaluable skill for later experiences outside the context of the immediate family or care situation.

Interacting with fathers and other secondary carers

Apart from participating in conversations with primary carers and siblings or slightly older children, infants also interact with secondary carers, often their father, and with other unfamiliar adults. To what extent does 'level of familiarity' affect interaction and what is its effect on language learning?

Apparently the speech of primary and secondary carers to infants differs little in terms of the main characteristics of 'motherese'. However, differences do occur in the way they interact with infants. For example, because they usually spend less time with the child, fathers tend to have difficulty understanding early communicative acts and more often request clarification of a message. This provides opportunities for the child to modify utterances to improve intelligibility (Barton and Tomasello, 1994). Fathers are also more demanding than mothers, asking more open-ended questions that require more than a yes/no response, resulting in the children producing more words when interacting with their fathers (Masur, 1997). In addition, the child learns that some conversational partners do not understand what they say and repetition or some other adjustment or elaboration may be needed. This experience helps children to acquire more intelligible and conventional forms of speech that will enhance their communication with adults who are even less familiar. Overall, fathers and siblings interacting with young children who are in the early stages of language acquisition are:

- less conversationally responsive, ignoring more often the child's linguistic overtures
- less conversationally supportive, providing the child with fewer conversation-maintaining devices such as questions and turnabouts
- less conversationally competent with the child in the sense that they experience more breakdowns, fewer successful repairs, and overall shorter conversations
- more directive of the topic of the conversation and the child's behaviour.

(Source: Barton and Tomasello, 1994, p. 133).

Helping slow, non-initiating and passive children

The importance of 'responsiveness' has been a recurring theme in the discussion on how adults interact with young language-learning children. Children who are passive and seldom initiate an activity or sound will need special help. This is a very difficult situation for parents, because lack of response from a child can be interpreted by a carer as a lack of communication, leading to the carer identifying fewer meanings in the infant's behaviour (Sapp, 2001). For example, infants with visual impairments are unable, or have limited ability, to use looking and pointing to achieve joint reference with a carer as effectively as infants with normal sight. They are also slower to begin to explore their environment, crawling and walking at a later age than their peers with normal vision (Ferrell, 1998). These delays can have a negative impact on the development of alternative, non-visual means of communication. There is also a risk that inadequate responsivity in infants will lead to carers spending less time with these children. In this situation, carers need to use the same strategies that are used with very young infants. These include:

- taking both roles in the interaction when carrying out the daily routines of dressing, bathing, feeding and so on
- talking about the immediate situation
- attracting the child's attention to noisy toys, coloured mobiles, moving leaves, trains going by and so on
- providing appropriate cues for communication and responding positively to any cues the child provides
- repeating or imitating and sounds, gestures or actions and encouraging the child to join in while respecting the child's pace
- allowing time for the child to respond
- ensuring that the child is motivated to respond
- extending the child's responses through 'scaffolding' to produce more complex responses.

It is not always possible to understand the reasons that underlie passivity in some children, particularly during periods of play. It has been suggested that environmental factors such as involvement in highly structured, adult-directed intervention, and biological factors such as delayed development in cognitive and motor skills, may contribute to reduced cognitive focus on an activity, slow responses and passivity (Hill and McCune-Nicolich, 1981; Cichetti and Ganiban, 1990). Periods of passivity during play may also be associated with the need for a break from activity (Cherkes-Julkowski and Gertner, 1989), an expectation that inactivity will lead to adult intervention and support (Goodman, 1992) or simply a low state of arousal or the need for time to pause and re-energize (Linn, Goodman and Lender, 2000).

Strategies for helping children who are slow or passive to encourage more active and responsive behaviour can begin with careful observation to identify situations where the child is most responsive, as well as those in which the child is most passive, how long this behaviour persists and what follows such episodes (Linn, Goodman and Lender, 2000). This information can then be used to engage the child's attention and heighten interest by carefully matching environmental conditions to the particular response patterns of the child (Bricker, 1992). Passivity and non-initiation can reflect different needs in different children. Care needs to be taken to balance efforts to stimulate greater responsiveness with respect for the particular needs and personal rhythm of each child.

Specific strategies for interacting with language-learning children are set out in 'Talking with children' in Appendix F.

Summary

During the period when they are acquiring language skills, children need responsive parents or carers who are quick to identify opportunities for interaction, and sensitive to the level that the child has reached in learning to communicate. The need for such interactive experiences is particularly important for children who are slow to talk. For these children, the scaffolding that primary and secondary carers provide is particularly important. Adults cannot 'teach' language to children but they can provide an optimal learning environment through contingent reciprocal interaction that continues throughout a sometimes extended period of language learning.

Part 2
Designing and implementing a language programme

In the following six chapters (5–10), guidelines are set out for designing and organizing a language programme for a child who needs help in the early stages of language development. Chapter 5 provides a general overview of the procedures to be followed in establishing a language intervention programme. Chapters 6–9 focus on the five programme levels described in Chapter 2 (see Table 2.1). These begin with the preliminary skills of shared attention and joint activity, and progress to the more complex skills of combining words into sentences, expressing ideas about possession and tense, and asking and answering questions. The first two components of language identified in Chapter 1 are also explored in these chapters: *meaning* or the intended topic of communication (semantics) and *rules* or the grammatical system that defines ways of combining words meaningfully (syntax and morphology). The *use* of language to communicate meaning (pragmatics) is examined in Chapter 10. Speech *sounds*, the mechanism by which meaning is conveyed to others (phonology), is considered in the first chapter of Part 3, Chapter 11.

The aim of the chapters in Parts 2 and 3 is to provide a very practical description of procedures that can be used to help children with problems in the early stages of communication development. Information in these chapters is presented in a direct and highly personal style, with the expectation that this will make the ideas more readily accessible to the reader. Remember that these suggestions are intended for use by teachers specializing in early childhood and special education, or carers, speech and language pathologists and therapists and parents who have the support of a professional.

Chapter 5
Organizing a language programme

In this chapter, we consider the steps that need to be taken if you want to help a child begin to communicate more effectively. First, you need to watch and listen to the child, to find out exactly how he or she is currently communicating. You also need to identify culturally appropriate activities and toys or other materials that the child enjoys. With this information, you can begin to select some appropriate language goals and plan activities for teaching. By the end of this chapter, you should have ideas on ways to find out exactly how the child is communicating now, examples of specific language teaching goals and activities that might be suitable for teaching new communication skills, and where and when your teaching activities could be carried out.

But before beginning to talk about actually planning and implementing a language programme, it is a good idea to review the basic principles or assumptions upon which the ideas used in the programme are based. These principles are derived from the interactional view of language learning described in Chapter 1.

Basic principles underlying the language programme

It is sometimes difficult to identify all of the basic principles that underlie programmes such as that described here. Some can be stated readily but others may not be obvious even to those closely involved in the programme. In thinking about the procedures that comprise the programme, six major principles can be identified:

- First words emerge as a result of children's daily experiences with people, objects and events.
- Children acquire language through interaction with consistent carers, at first parents, then other family members, teachers and others.
- When children have difficulty in learning to talk, experiences can be provided that will encourage their language development.

- Language activities are best carried out in children's natural setting with familiar adults.
- New and emerging skills need to be practised frequently, whenever opportunities arise throughout the day, with clear speech models provided by interactive partners to ensure that the children learn to associate specific speech sounds with their actions.
- Preliminary skills including attending, turn-taking and imitation need to be acquired. Appropriate play skills are also required, since first words will emerge out of children's play activities.

The programme described in this book is based on the assumption that children learn to talk by engagement with their environment and interaction with responsive others. Central to this process is the active role taken by the children themselves, who must make sense of these experiences. Cognitive, social and affective processes are involved. The content of the language programme is derived from aspects of the environment that interest children. A linguistic system is also involved in that children must learn the language of their community. The programme is, therefore, based on three main components:

- children's active participation in social exchanges
- children's knowledge of the physical world and the relationship of objects and actions within it
- children's gradual acquisition of a shared system of symbols that can be used to communicate meaning to others.

The remaining sections of this chapter give an outline of the general procedures that you should follow to help a specific child who is having difficulties in the development of early language skills. Specific details of assessment methods and intervention strategies are described in Chapters 6–10.

How to set up a language programme

It is a good idea to begin by collecting information about the child's current communicative behaviour. This process is sometimes called 'screening'. Here your aim is to collect simple information, using quick methods, as a first step in identifying the skills that the child has already acquired. Once you have collected this information, you can begin to assess the child more carefully and plan an intervention programme.

Initial screening of current communication skills

The best way to find out how a child is communicating is by observation. You will also need to write down examples of what is said or done. You can do this by watching the child carefully in everyday situations. You may also need to give the child a set of tasks that provide an opportunity to demonstrate current skills. Ask significant others who spend time with the child, including parents, teachers and other carers, to help you collect this information.

Here are some examples of the kind of information that you could collect. Remember to note what the child does and says, and the context in which this occurs.

- How does the child attract your attention?
- How does the child tell you something important, such as 'Daddy is coming'?
- How does the child tell you what he has found, or is doing or looking at?
- How does the child tell you that she is hungry, or cold?
- How does the child tell you other interesting things?

Try to collect up to 10 examples of the way that the child communicates this type of information. Write down what the child does or says as exactly as you can. If some of the child's words are not clear, write the sounds that the child makes. Then write the word that you think the child is trying to say in brackets beside the sounds, just to remind yourself of what you think the child wants to say.

Taking a language sample

Another way to find out how a child is communicating is to collect a sample of language or other communication skills. To do this, you need to make a tape- or video-recording of you or another person playing with the child. Try to record at least 10 minutes' play. Use some toys or picture books that the child likes. The adult should try not to talk too much during the session. The aim is to encourage the child to talk. You can replay the tape or video later and write down exactly what the child said or did. Try to collect at least 20 utterances, whether they are gestures, sounds or words. Guidelines for taking a language sample are set out in Appendix A.

Once you have collected some information about how the child is communicating now, you will be able to work out what level of language development he or she has reached. The material you have collected will also be useful when you begin to plan a programme, as a source of ideas about the actions, sounds or words that you can begin to teach.

Identifying what the child likes to do

When you begin to plan ways to help a child learn to talk, you need to identify some of the activities, games and toys that the child is very interested in or enjoys. Children need to feel relaxed and confident in any activity that they share with you. They need to feel that the activity is fun and that they are taking part because they want to, not because you expect them to. It will be easier for you to engage their attention if you select something that you know will attract and hold their attention.

Here are some examples of activities that most children enjoy:

- games with a ball
- playing with blocks and model cars and trains
- drawing
- games with dolls and soft toys
- looking at books
- going for a walk or driving in the car
- doing jigsaw puzzles
- running, hiding
- tea parties
- preparing food and eating
- talking.

Watch the child and make a list of the activities, toys or events that he or she particularly enjoys. Try to find activities that are associated with different times of the day and with different locations, such as during quiet times after waking up from a sleep, after tea, during the bath if it is not too hectic, outside in the garden, at the park and so on. Also think about the types of toys that interest the child, such as balls, model cars, soft toys and dolls, books about trains, wind-up toys. Make a list of about five activities and objects that might be appropriate for using in language games. This will give you ideas about the contexts in which you can practise language skills. You will also know which materials will engage the child's attention. You will now need to assemble any equipment that you plan to use. A list of the materials that parents and others have found to be useful in engaging children's interest in language games is given in Table 5.1.

Identifying the appropriate language level

Once you have observed the child and collected information about how he or she is communicating now, and any preferred activities and toys, you can decide the programme level that you think the child has reached. Ideas for more detailed assessment of children's current communication skills are given in Chapters 6–9. Each of these chapters is concerned with a particular programme level, and you need to decide which chapter is likely to be most relevant for any particular child. For example, if the child is not yet using consistent gestures, sounds or words you should turn to programme level 1 (Chapter 6) which is concerned with the preliminary skills of looking together, turn-taking and imitation, and appropriate play. If the child has these early skills but does not use intelligible words, you should begin with level 2 (Chapter 7). If the child is just beginning to produce single words, turn to level 3 (Chapter 8). If the child is beginning to put two words together, look at level 4 or, perhaps, level 5 (Chapter 9).

Table 5.1 The essential collection (toys and other useful teaching resources for children at all levels of development)

Balls, blocks of all sizes and shapes, cars, planes
Simple train set or something similar
Model farm or zoo animals and people
Cups, bowls, spoons, tea pot, cooking utensils
Playdough, rollers, cutters
Containers; all sizes and shapes to use as a bath, washing up bowl, small bucket, etc.
Clothes, face washers
Teddy, soft dolls with removable clothes
Bed and bed clothes; cardboard box or cushion for a doll's bed
Old clothes, nappies/diapers, hats
Glove or finger puppets
Purses, bags, boxes of all sizes for objects to be put in and taken out
A postbox or 'gone' box Large cardboard boxes in which a child can sit
Noise-makers; xylophone, bells, shakers, drum and so forth
Simple puzzles
Picture books; make your own from photo albums, plastic folders clipped together, magazines, old cards and so on (involve other members of family in making these)
Paper and crayons for drawing
Junk; for example, plastic bottles, empty spools, cotton reels, scraps of cloth (use your imagination)
Mirror
Surprise bag (small cloth bag with drawstring or elastic around the top; opening big enough to allow child to feel what is inside and pull objects out)
Jack-in-the-box, musical toy
Tapes of music; bought or make your own of music and songs that the child enjoys

For children with more advanced skills
Lottos, dominos, colour matching games and so on
Early reading books

Issues associated with appropriate use of language (communicative intentions) are considered in Chapter 10. You should refer to this information at the same time as you begin to work on one of the programme levels, since development in pragmatic skills increases at the same time as other aspects of language development. Each chapter begins with suggestions for more detailed assessment of the child's language skills in the particular aspect of language that is the focus of that chapter. Summary assessment sheets to assist you in recording the child's skills at each level are included in Appendix B.

When selecting an appropriate level at which to begin, you need to remember that it is advisable to start at a point where the child will experience success. This will help to ensure that the child enjoys interacting with you and cooperates in your planned activities. Look at the language level that the child is at now, as a starting point for your programme, rather than moving too quickly to a level where he or she is likely to experience difficulties and lose interest in your games.

Selecting language objectives

You can select some initial teaching objectives from information obtained from assessment of the child. These will comprise the specific actions, gestures, sounds, words or simple sentences that you have decided the child could learn. How will you decide what to teach the child? A number of factors are important in choosing teaching objectives. Who are the most important people in the child's life? Are there favourite games or events? Is there a security blanket or similar favourite object? What does the child like to eat or drink? There are unlimited possibilities for topics from which you can select items to teach, but it is important that the ones you choose are appropriate for this particular child. They will help the child move to a higher level of language functioning.

It is usually appropriate that you select four or five actions, gestures, sounds, words or phrases as your first teaching objectives. Later, when you and the child are familiar with the new routine, this list can be extended to include 10 items. At the start of a programme, it is a good idea to include a few items that you suspect the child already knows. We call these 'success' items. They help to make the child feel good about taking part in the programme and be willing to participate in your planned activities. Once you begin, you will need to monitor progress in the items you have chosen. Those that are learned can be dropped from the list and new items selected. Those that are not learned will also need to be replaced with other items that may be more successful. Details about the implementation of this process are described in the following five chapters.

Planning where, when and how to implement language activities

Now you have decided what to teach and which activities to use in your teaching you need to plan where the teaching will take place and at what time or times of the day. You will also have to think about how you will introduce the activities. What role will you take? Answers to these questions will be determined by the specific goals and activities that you have chosen. For example, words associated with water, taps and washing will be taught at bathtime and, if you have time and are patient enough, while you are washing up or sweeping the floor. Words to do with eating are best taught at meal or snack-times. Some of your teaching should be carried out, if possible, during special times that you set aside to spend with the child. You will need to choose a time when you and the child will be fairly free from other distractions and a place where you will both be comfortable. If necessary, you might have to organize activities to occupy other children while you are busy, though they can often be included in your activity (see Chapter 14). Or you may be able to find a time when others are already well occupied.

In developing a plan for teaching the child, you will need to decide when, where and how you will implement these ideas:

When?   In the morning, after tea, before bed
Where? In the kitchen, the garden
How?   While sitting on the floor playing with a car, having a tea party or getting ready to go outside.

Language teaching is best carried out in three types of situations:

* within daily routines
* at appropriate times that occur spontaneously during the day
* as part of planned activities that have a high level of interest for the child.

Much of children's learning occurs during routine events. These types of situations recur often and have a predictable format or script (see Chapter 3). Examples include:

* eating lunch
* washing up
* reading a book
* playing on outside equipment
* putting away the blocks
* going for a rest.

Within the relatively fixed set of activities associated with these types of events, opportunities should be planned for children to practise appropriate language skills. For example, level 1 turn-taking can be practised while rolling a ball, saying 'my turn', 'your turn'. Level 2 performative sounds such as 'whee' and 'oo-oo' can be practised on a swing. There are many opportunities for using the single words and simple sentences of levels 3 and 4 during mealtimes, as when the adult says 'do you want egg or tomato?' and the child replies 'egg'. On family visits, the child can practise saying 'hello Nana', 'hello Auntie' or count the stairs 'one, two, three, four'. The more advanced skills of level 5 can be practised while shopping, with the child asking questions about what is needed and describing what has been bought. It is important to take advantage of these recurring situations because they provide a rich source of opportunities for children to practise simple language skills. Similarly, nursery rhymes and familiar stories with repeated dialogue such as *The Three Bears* and the *Three Billy Goats Gruff* also allow children to practise talking.

Many opportunities for teaching language occur spontaneously during the day. For example, the child at level 1 can be encouraged to imitate Mummy clapping her hands or drinking tea. Skills such as waving good-bye can be learned when someone leaves or arrives. Performative sounds such as 'br'mm' and 'toot toot' can be practised when going for a ride in a bus or a car, and 'woof' and 'pr'rr' or 'miaou' when the child sees a dog or a cat. Single words, simple sentences and more advanced skills can be practised, while unpacking a shopping bag or going for a walk. These kinds of situations are particularly appropriate if language-teaching experiences can only be provided within normal daily activities, either at home or in an early childhood group setting.

Planned activities that are highly interesting to the child can be used to practise language. For example, for the child at level 1 in the language programme, activities involving blocks, pop-up toys, puppets, finger plays and 'boo' games are a good way to teach the preliminary skills of looking and attending, taking turns, imitation and appropriate play. At level 2, activities with dolls or soft toys, small cars, model animals and musical instruments provide opportunities to encourage performative sounds such as 'br'mm', 'moo' and 'bang'. Matching objects to pictures is a good way to encourage a child at level 3 to label these objects, and games such as lotto or snap are useful for teaching the level 4 and 5 skills of early sentences and asking questions.

To be successful, the same games are usually repeated over a number of days or weeks. This gives the child time to learn the skills that have been selected for teaching. Often, three or four different games are included in each practice session, with new games introduced and old ones discarded according to the interest and progress of the child. Children need time to learn and then enjoy repeating familiar activities and playing with favourite objects over and over again.

Playing with children

If you are not used to sitting and playing with the child, or if you are a little unsure about how to begin, here are some suggestions about ways of sharing in games, encouraging play and introducing new toys. You should remember that, for many children, the world is very big and threatening; they like to be close to a carer for security and support. Children will be happy that you are near and showing an interest in what they are doing. Sharing the game will give you both a sense of closeness.

If you find it difficult to begin a game with the child, try starting off by just sitting nearby. Get down on the floor if you possibly can. If this feels strange, try sitting down with something to occupy you such as a book or some work. Give the child some toys to play with, and when he is happily involved with the toys, you can look at what he is doing. The child will just be happy to have you near, and watching. In time, the child will come close to you, perhaps showing you a toy. Then you can comment on the toy or on what the child is doing. Before you know it, you will have begun to follow the child's lead and joined in the game. You still need to remember to stop, sometimes, to watch and listen to the child as he plays. Once this joint attention is established, you will be in a position to guide and extend the child in the game. At this stage, your smiles and laughter will tell the child that you approve. In this way you build up the child's confidence.

If a child seems to lose interest in an activity, you might find that this is a good time to introduce some simple songs and rhymes. You can change the words of the songs to suit what you are doing, incorporating key words or sounds that you want to teach into your song ('This is the way we roll the ball', for example).

When you and the child are comfortable sitting together and playing, you can start introducing new toys and actions as well as the new ways of using familiar toys; feeding and bathing teddy, building a bridge for the cars and pushing them through it, rolling the ball back and forth. These simple routines will encourage the child to take turns with you in a game, and help to develop new play skills. Do not expect the child to follow all your ideas. Encourage the child when she discovers new ways of doing things without your help. Remember, as you play, to comment on what both you and the child are doing, and to use appropriate noises and gestures or words during the game, such as 'br'mm', 'boo', 'gone' and so on.

At this stage, it is also important to have a variety of things to play with so that the child can choose what is most interesting. These items need not be expensive: blocks, balls, old containers into which things can be put to roll and shake, cardboard boxes and kitchen utensils are all interesting to children. It is a good idea to have a box or cupboard where the child can have ready access to the toys and be free to explore. New items can be added from time to time and broken items, or those that no longer interest the child, can be removed. Simple toys are best. By sticking to simple toys that the child can easily manipulate, you will avoid or lessen the inevitable frustration that comes with a toy that breaks too easily or is too difficult or complicated.

If possible, you should try to select language objectives to practise in all of the situations described here. If it is too difficult to include a special playtime in your daily routine, make sure you look for appropriate opportunities during the day and try to identify some regular event where a relevant language task can be practised.

If you cannot provide individual sessions and must incorporate your language teaching into an early childhood context that involves groups of children, then the routine situations described here are particularly important as a means to teaching appropriate language skills to a child. Moreover, once you know the objectives that are appropriate, you can include specific language goals for each of the children involved in a group activity. For example, at snack and drink times, or when asking for equipment or permission to go outside, children can be taught to use appropriate actions, gestures, sounds or words to get what they want or need. Group situations have the advantage that each child can see and hear peers model appropriate actions and speech. This issue is discussed in more detail in Chapter 14.

Involving all the family

Finally, you should try to involve the whole family in your language programme. At home, ensure that everyone knows what you are doing and
has an opportunity to join in. Older brothers and sisters are often interested and have time to help when parents are unable or too busy. All
those involved with the child need to be told about your current language
objectives. This will help to ensure that the child is encouraged to use any
new skills at every opportunity.

Once the child begins to use the new skills that you have been teaching, tell others such as grandparents, aunts and uncles and the babysitter
what the child has learned to do. At home, write it on a card and tape it
on the refrigerator. Write a note to the preschool teacher or other helpers,
so that they can encourage the child to use the new skills at appropriate
times. Some parents, teachers and carers find it useful to keep a record of
what they are working on and how the child is progressing in a communication or language book. Such a book provides a good source of
information for everyone who is helping the child or is interested in his
progress. Involving everyone in the programme ensures plenty of practice
with different people. This will help the child to progress more quickly to
the next level in the language programme.

Checking progress

Once you have begun to implement some specific teaching objectives you
will need to carry out some form of evaluation to check whether or not
your objectives have been achieved. Here, you will be interested in
progress on specific objectives, and progress on programme levels.

Progress on specific objectives

Sometimes it is helpful to monitor a child's progress on a current language objective by noting at regular intervals whether a particular action
or sound is produced successfully by the child. If you wish to record this
information formally, the observation record forms in Appendix C can
be used for this purpose. These sheets are most appropriate if you are
using planned games in your language programme. Video-recording an
activity can also be helpful because it enables you to check how the
child is progressing, particularly when you do not have time to record
what is happening during a game and find it difficult to remember what
happened later. This type of information is useful in two ways. It is helpful as a means of deciding when to move on to a new activity or higher
level in the language programme. It can also help you realize that the
child is learning the skill you want to teach, and this can be important
if progress is slow. Very slow progress may result from the child's lack of

interest in the activity you have chosen, or because the task is too difficult. In either case, you may need to abandon that activity and choose
another one.

Progress on programme levels

When a child appears to be quickly learning the tasks you have planned,
without much practice, you should find out if it is time to move on to the
next level in the language programme. To check the child's progress, you
can reuse the tasks you gave the child initially or find a similar set to check
on current skills.

Once you have assessed the child and know the level of his or her current skills, you can begin to plan your teaching programme. Details of
planning at each language level are set out in Chapters 6–10.

Hints for setting up a successful language programme for a child

Assessment

- Take time to assess the child's current language competence before you
  start. This will ensure that you have identified the appropriate level to
  begin teaching. Several periods of both formal and informal observation are better than one long period.
- Seek information about the child's communication abilities, styles and
  strategies from relevant adults, including parents, other family members, teachers and other carers. Ask about how the child communicates
  with them.

Selecting teaching objectives

- Identify at least one activity that interests the child. This will be the context in which you will implement your objectives.
- Think of four or five actions, sounds or words to introduce within the
  activity you have selected. These will be the specific items that you will
  plan to teach. Include at least one or two that the child can already do
  as 'success' items. Note that in some cases, such as when the aim is to
  encourage the child to look at something of interest with you (see the
  early part of Chapter 6), the specific objective will be 'looking together'. Here, your goal will not involve identifying specific sounds or
  words to teach.
- Choose achievable targets at first. Do not worry if some appear too
  easy. They will give you the opportunity to provide lots of praise and
  allow the child to experience success. You can always move on quickly,
  once you and the child have become accustomed to the procedure.

This is much better than letting the child become 'stuck' on difficult targets.

- Do not be worried about dropping an unsuccessful item. It may not have been appropriate or of interest to the child at the time you introduced it. If it is one you would like her to achieve, try it again later after the child has experienced success with other items.

Organizing a practice session

- Decide how to set up the activity to ensure that there are opportunities for the planned words or actions to occur.
- Collect the materials you will need. Try to keep them ready to use when a suitable opportunity arises. Make sure you are organized before you invite the child to play with you.
- Introduce only a few new target items at a time. Initially, both you and the child will need to learn the rules of the new game. Once you have developed your relationship within the activity, the child's communication behaviour will tell you when it is time to introduce some new items.
- Choose targets that are easy for you to implement. In particular, they should interest the child and be relevant to his or her needs.
- Remember to provide ample opportunity for the child to practise with as many people as possible in a variety of situations. Several short sessions lasting 5–10 minutes are better than one long session. However, periods of play and routine activities usually provide the best times to practise. Make as much use as possible of opportunities that arise spontaneously during the day.
- Give lots of praise. Young children respond well to a quick hug, a smile and the sound of pleasure in your voice.
- Slip in occasional opportunities to practise recently learned items in your current play to ensure that they are maintained. Practice is the key to retention of newly acquired skills.

Involving family and friends

- Make sure that everyone who has contact with the child, including parents, siblings, other family members, teachers, the babysitter and other carers, know about your current goals. Encourage them to practise these goals with the child if there is an appropriate opportunity. Use a communication or language book to let others know what you are doing and encourage them to keep you informed about anything relevant. Put notes on the refrigerator and family or staff notice boards to remind relevant adults about your current goals. Other ideas are included in Chapter 14.
- If the child has interested siblings or friends, encourage them to become involved. It is amazing what a child can learn from another

more competent child. This also helps overcome difficulties that are sometimes encountered when one child appears to get more adult attention than others do. The 'helper' will be rewarded by the attention given to this 'helpfulness'.

Selecting new goals and moving on to the next programme level

- Once the child shows that an item has been learned – being able to tap the table and say 'bang' on three separate occasions, for example – drop this item from your list. Choose a new task. Refer to the following chapters for criteria to use when deciding the time to move from one language level to the next.
- If the child does not appear to be learning a particular item that you have been practising for at least two weeks, you may need to reconsider its interest or difficulty level. It might be appropriate to replace that item with a new one.
- At all times, avoid confronting a child with demands to 'look', 'do' or 'say'. The child will usually try to join in your tasks if they are embedded in an interesting activity or game. If the child does not want to join in, you may need to change your plans. Perhaps the activity is not interesting, or the child may not like sitting with you. You may need to look for naturally occurring situations in which to embed the practice. The tasks you have selected may be too difficult and you may need to move back to an earlier level in the programme, to establish the new routine. Above all, make your language activities fun for both you and the child.
- The most important points to remember when you begin to practise language tasks are to follow the child's lead, ask only three times and avoid confrontation.

Summary

In this chapter, suggestions are made about the steps that you will need to take before you can begin to help a child learn new language skills. Strategies are outlined to find out how a child is currently communicating, what the child's main interests are, which teaching goals to select and how to set about achieving these goals.

In the next chapter, specific ideas are given for helping children who lack the preliminary skills of looking together, turn-taking and imitation, and appropriate play. Subsequent chapters in this part of the book focus on the preverbal skills of performatives and protowords, and then first words and beyond. Each of these chapters describes ways to assess a child. Suggestions are then made for selecting and practising appropriate language and communication goals. Practical ideas for a variety of suitable activities and games are included here. Finally, each chapter ends with suggestions about how to decide when it is time to move on to the next level in the language programme.

Chapter 6
Preliminary skills:
programme level 1

The sounds that an infant makes are important precursors of language and, in particular, later phonological development, but babbling does not lead directly to speech. First words are derived from the child's earliest experiences with objects and, more particularly, with people. So if children are delayed in learning to talk, attention needs to be paid to their daily activities and their interaction with familiar people and objects. In this chapter, suggestions are made about ways to find out if a child has acquired three of the key skills that are needed to interact with people and objects. These include the skills of looking at something of interest with an adult (this is sometimes called 'joint attention' or 'shared gaze'), taking turns in an activity, and knowing how to play appropriately with a variety of objects and materials. The chapter is divided into three sections, each of which is concerned with one of these three key skills. Each section includes details of procedures to assess a child's performance in the focus skill. Practical suggestions are then made about activities and materials that can be used with the child to improve performance in the target skill. Assistance is given on ways to check the child's progress and decide when to move on to the next task.

Research evidence suggests that language development is dependent on three major types of experiences involving both people and objects:

- *Looking together or joint attention* – learning to look at something interesting with an adult, such as a butterfly, the moon or a picture of a puppy.
- *Turn-taking* – learning to take turns with an adult in a shared activity. This involves imitation, which is a powerful means of helping a child to acquire and practise the skills needed to take part in a conversation. It might involve learning to take turns with a special toy, or imitate actions to wave 'goodbye'.
- *Appropriate play* – the acquisition of strategies needed to explore and manipulate the variety of objects and materials that children encounter each day, such as learning to push a toy car or build a tower from blocks.

Children can learn these skills in any order, but they need to learn to look at something interesting with another person first. Some children begin to play appropriately before they learn to imitate or take turns. However, these three skills are important if a child is to learn to communicate effectively. So, whatever the language level of the child, you will need to check each of these areas and be prepared to give more practice if these skills seem to be lacking.

Looking together

In Chapter 2, we reviewed research on the sequence of levels that children pass through as they learn to talk (Bloom, 1970; Brown, 1973; Halliday, 1975; Bates, 1976). These studies suggested that the origins of communication lie in activities that involve the child and an adult in jointly attending to objects and events that interest them both. Check if this child will follow your lead and look at things with you.

Assessment of looking-together skills

The main goal here is to find out if the child can follow your lead to look at something. You can check these skills by observing the child at different times during the day. Alternatively, you can set up a special time and check the child's responses to selected activities. Here are some ideas to check these skills. Notice that the four activities described here range from relatively simple tasks such as looking at a colourful toy to the more difficult task of looking at a book with an adult. You should substitute other similar activities if you feel those suggested here are not appropriate for this child. Your aim is to find out if the child has the skills identified here.

Whatever activities you decide to use, remember to allow enough time for the child to respond to each task. Some children react very slowly and you need to allow them enough time to respond. You might be able to record the assessment with a video-recorder. You can then check the child's responses more carefully later. You can use the summary assessment sheet for preliminary skills in Appendix B to record the results of the assessment.

Suggested assessment activities

- Will the child look at an interesting toy that is put in front of her? Find a toy that moves, makes a sound or is colourful, such as a jack-in-the-box or pull-along toy with moving parts that makes a noise. Encourage the child to watch it. Does the child look at the toy for at least 5 seconds?
- Will the child look at a paper bag in which you have hidden a surprise? Hide a small toy, such as a ball, in a paper bag. Attract the child's attention and make sure that he knows something is hidden in the bag. Open the bag slowly and let the child find the toy. Does the child look at what is happening for at least 5 seconds?

- Will the child look at your hands while you play a finger game or a hiding game with a favourite soft toy? Sing a nursery rhyme that has hand movements, such as 'Twinkle Twinkle Little Star' or 'Open, Shut Them'. Play a game with a favourite toy; first hiding it and then letting it appear gradually or suddenly. Does the child look for at least 5 seconds?
- Will the child look at pictures or a book with you? Take a favourite book, one with clear simple pictures. You could also use pictures cut out of magazines and pasted into a scrapbook, or a photo album with pictures of the family. Sit beside the child and look at the pictures in the book, talking about them and pointing at anything of interest. Does the child look at most of the pictures that you point to for at least 5 seconds?

If the child attends to three or four of the activities, you can assume that he or she has the target skill and can move on to the next task. A child who is able to do only one or two of the four tasks probably needs to practise very simple looking-together activities.

Suggestions for practising looking-together skills

Think of a number of activities that are likely to interest the child and provide opportunities for developing looking-together skills. These could include playing with interesting toys, finger rhymes, games with puppets or looking at simple, colourful picture books. Remember that you can repeat a game that interests the child several times during one practice session and over several days, or until you think the child is beginning to lose interest. Stop well before the child is bored.

Play these practice games with the child sitting close beside you or on your lap. If appropriate, try to keep the activity close to your face and exaggerate your facial gestures so that the child learns to look at your face as well as the toy. Keep the toy under your control and close to you. Look at the child and, as appropriate, talk about the toy's colour, movement and sound. Give the child plenty of time to react to what is happening and respond positively when the child looks at the toy. Your aim is to teach the child to look with you at an interesting object or event.

Interesting toys

Most children enjoy and will watch toys that move, make a sound and are colourful. Here are some suggestions for such toys:

- balls
- favourite soft toys
- Jack-in-the-box or pop-up toys
- wind-up or pull-along toys
- toys with moveable parts: a bus with people inside, a fire engine with crane or a garage with opening doors

- blocks: build a tower and knock it over, build a tunnel
- model cars: cars that make a noise, trains
- model animals: fences, people
- water and sand play: pouring, splashing, patting
- play dough: rolling, squashing, cutting
- musical instruments: banging, shaking.

Finger games and nursery rhymes

Try to choose songs and rhymes that are brief and interesting for a child who is not yet able to attend for long. Make the actions near your face to encourage the child to look at your lips and eyes, or play a finger game that involves touching some part of the child's body. Sit on the floor with the child beside you in front of a mirror. Do the actions with your hands beside the child. You can use any favourite family songs. Your aim is to do the songs and rhymes together, with the child watching and listening. You can use any songs or rhymes that you know the child enjoys. Here are some examples of suitable songs and rhymes:

- Twinkle, Twinkle Little Star
- Incy Wincy Spider
- This Little Piggy
- Round and Round The Garden
- Open, Shut Them
- Roly Poly.

Puppets

Simple but attractive puppets can be made out of old socks. Put your fingers in the toes of the sock and bend your fingers to touch the heel, to open and shut the puppet's mouth. Or draw faces on the inside of your fingers. Bend and dance your fingers to accompany a song. Most children are fascinated by the movements and sounds made by puppets, which can be a powerful means of drawing their attention to you.

Pictures and books

Looking with a child at pictures and books is a very effective way for a child to practise attending closely to an activity with an adult. This is also a time when the language that the adult uses with the child is important. Remember that Chapter 4 and Appendix F set out clear guidelines on how to talk to children so that they hear good models of appropriate language.

When selecting books for language development experiences, begin with very simple picture books that have clear illustrations of familiar objects such as an apple, cup, keys, chair, plate, spoon and shoe. Books can be made to suit children's particular interests by cutting pictures from magazines and pasting them into a scrapbook or mounting them in picture albums. Family photos can also be used. Albums have the advantage that the pictures can be changed as the child's interests change. Use albums with pages that are strong enough to be handled often by a child.

While looking at books, point to anything that is likely to interest the child, commenting with clear simple words. Allow time for the child to look and respond. Remember that children with poor skills need many more opportunities than other children to practise a new task, so look at the same book or set of pictures for as long as the child remains interested.

Taking the next step

When should you decide to move on to the next skill? You need to check to see if the child is progressing in the tasks you have been practising. Select at least two toys and two finger plays that are not familiar to the child. See if the child will attend to them for at least 5 seconds when you show them. If the child does not watch at least three items you need to give more practice. If the child watches three of the four items, it is probably time to move on to the next section.

Turn-taking and imitation

Turn-taking and imitation are two important skills that underlie learning to talk. Both these skills reflect the social bases of language. Learning to speak involves not only understanding the meaning of words and how to produce them, but also when to talk and how to take turns in a conversation. Imitation is important because it is a means for the child to learn how to produce words. So if children are to acquire effective language skills, they need to learn how to take turns with a partner and how to imitate what the partner is doing and saying. Some children who can talk still need practice in turn-taking skills so that they can begin to use the words they know to communicate effectively.

Initially, turn-taking and imitation skills are learned through games that involve the child in cooperative activities with an adult. Including a sound in the game (for example, when playing 'Boo' or 'Boomps-a-Daisy') gives the child an opportunity to imitate both actions and sounds. Eventually, the sound rather than the action part of the activity becomes significant for the child. This is discussed in more detail in the next chapter (Chapter 7).

Does your child know how to take turns and imitate what a partner in a game does? Here are some suggestions for checking these skills. Note that if the child is unable to do one of the suggested tasks, you should give some practice and repeat the task. This strategy (test–practice–test) is followed because it is important to know if the child is able to learn from even a very brief practice session. A child who is ready to acquire these skills will probably respond to more practice. If there is no change in skill levels after some practice, it is likely that the child is not yet ready to learn these skills.

Assessment of turn-taking and imitation skills

You can assess a child's skills in turn-taking and imitation by observing him or her carefully during appropriate daily activities, or by setting up a series of tasks. Here are some suggestions for assessing these skills. Substitute alternative activities if you feel these suggestions are not appropriate for the child. Use the relevant summary sheet in Appendix B to record your results.

Suggested assessment activities

Turn-taking

- Will the child join in a game with you that involves taking turns with a toy? Sit opposite the child on the floor or at a table. Push a toy car towards the child, roll a ball or throw a beanbag. Encourage the child to return the object to you. Does the child return the object? If not, provide some practice: model the task again and encourage the child to take a turn in the game. Now re-administer the task. Does the child take a turn after practice?
- Will the child take turns with you in an activity involving objects? Sit opposite the child with an activity that includes small parts that can easily be put in/on or taken out/off. Suitable activities include a collection of small blocks or other items that can be put into a container or a set of coloured pegs and a pegboard. Demonstrate an action. For example, take a block out of the container or a peg off the board. Say 'Look, my turn'. Model the action. Encourage the child to take a turn in the activity. Say 'Your turn' or '(child's name)'s turn'. Does the child take a turn in the game? If not, provide some practice and re-administer the task. Does the child take a turn after practice?

Imitation

- Will the child join in a game with you and imitate what you do? Hide your face with your hands and as you uncover your face, say 'boo'. Does the child copy you and hide, or allow you to help her hide and then reappear? If not, help her to imitate this action. Model the task again and encourage imitation by shaping her hands to imitate your actions. Now re-administer the task. Does the child do the action after practice?
- Will the child imitate simple actions that you model? Sit opposite the child. Select four simple actions, such as:
  – clap hands
  – hit table
  – rub tummy
  – drop a toy.

Model each action and encourage the child to imitate what you do. Does the child imitate the action? If not, give some practice. Model each action again and encourage the child to imitate you. Shape the hands. Now re-administer the task. Does the child imitate the action after practice?

If the child is able to do three or four items on the first attempt, including at least two imitation tasks, you can move on to the next section. A child who is only able to do one of the two actions after practice is probably not yet ready to begin these activities. If the child can do two or more items after practice, you should continue to practise these games.

Suggestions for practising turn-taking and imitation skills

Think of a number of activities that involve you and the child in taking turns and imitation. It is important to select activities that the child finds interesting and will enjoy repeating over several days. Remember that you have two goals:

- to teach the child to take turns
- to teach the child to imitate your actions.

Both these skills are very useful for helping the child to acquire good play skills, as well as for learning to talk. Remember to say 'my turn' and '(child's name)'s turn', so that the child learns the rules of the game. A physical prompt such as patting the child's hand may help. When you are teaching a new activity, always demonstrate it first before asking the child to imitate you. For example, if you want the child to build a three-block tower, say 'watch me' or 'look'. Then you build the tower. Give the blocks to the child and say 'now you do it'. If necessary, help the child to pick up a block and put it on top of another. When the child can do the activity with a model, then just say 'you build' or '(child's name) build'. Say 'my turn', 'your turn' if you want the game to include turn-taking. If the child has difficulty waiting for his turn, you may also find it useful to praise him with words and a gesture such as a pat on the arm or knee for 'good waiting'.

When selecting activities or actions for the child to learn to imitate, select a sound or word that you can pair with each action. For example, you can label each action or make an appropriate sound such as 'smack lips', 'yum yum', 'eat', 'drink', 'sleep', 'walk' during a game with a soft toy or doll. Alternatively, you can accompany an action such as rolling a ball or pushing a model car with a sound such as 'oh!' or 'br'mm br'mm'. This will allow the child to begin to associate particular sound patterns with specific actions or games, and will provide a basis for you to begin to teach early sounds (see Chapter 7) and words (see Chapter 8).

When introducing a new activity, you will need to first model appropriate actions and then encourage turn-taking and imitation. This can take place in situations that allow for relatively informal play, such as with water, or in a sandpit. Play these activities with the child close to you so that she can watch you easily. Model appropriate actions. Show the child what you are doing and encourage imitation. Say, 'Look, you do this' or 'Jilly's turn'. Some appropriate actions to imitate in informal turn-taking games include:

- soft toys and dolls: wash face, brush hair, set table, eat
- kitchen corner: cook dinner, pour tea, drink, wash up
- water play: pour, empty, fill, splash
- sand play: dig, fill bucket, build castle, make cakes
- dough: roll, pat, cut, pile up
- blocks: build tower and push over
- cars and trains: push cars down ramp, under bridge
- balls, small bean bags: put into bucket and empty out
- outside equipment: take turns on slippery dip, climb through tunnel
- mechanical toys: take turns to operate a wind-up toy
- commercial games: take turns with picture lotto.

Some examples of actions to imitate (sit opposite the child or in front of a mirror) include:

- Roly Poly with hands
- touch parts of the body: head, nose, lips, knees, toes
- shake hands: clap hands
- hammer fists together
- stamp feet
- touch finger to lips
- make a kissing noise
- bang two blocks together
- bang a drum or other musical instrument.

Action songs and games

Children usually enjoy action songs and will often produce appropriate sounds in such songs. Here are some suggestions for songs that are particularly appropriate to use in turn-taking and imitation activities. They are also useful if you are working with a child in a group situation (see also Chapter 14). Where the song can include a variety of actions let each child suggest what to do. Some examples of appropriate action songs include:

- Ring-A-Ring-A-Rosie
- Row, Row, Row Your Boat
- Here We Go Round the Mulberry Bush
- Everybody Do This
- The Wheels of the Bus
- Simon Says
- Five Little Ducks Went Out One Day.

Taking the next step

If you think the child has learned to take turns with you and imitate your actions, check by introducing four new activities that you have not already practised. If the child is able to do at least three, you can probably move on to the next section. Remember to provide plenty of opportunities to take turns during each day because you will base your teaching of first words on the skills the child acquires during turn-taking and imitation activities. If the child does not succeed in at least three items, you need to give more practice.

Appropriate play

Language emerges out of a child's experiences, particularly from those that involve actions with toys and objects, as well as people. For example, before using a word to represent an object, the child must have strategies for exploring and learning about the object. Initially, a baby will mouth an object, wave it, drop it and bang it, but over time these strategies are combined to become more complicated, as in waving and then dropping, or putting the object into a container. New ways of exploring objects are also learned, such as squeezing, biting, pushing, hiding or throwing. Sometimes a sound is added to an action sequence, for example, dropping it and saying 'oh-oh' or pushing it and saying 'br'mm'. Often these sounds have been heard by the child while playing the dropping game with a carer or a game of pushing cars with a sibling.

Over time, the child will begin to use a part of the game or familiar routine to indicate that she remembers it and wants to do it again. The remembered part could be a gesture (hand movements to represent pushing the car) or a sound ('br'mm'). Similar actions and sounds may be used to represent other daily routines in the child's life such as a grasping action to indicate that he wants a toy that is out of reach or showing a tumbler to indicate thirst. The significant point is that the child develops a repertoire of actions and sounds associated with daily experiences. This is the substance out of which words emerge.

Assessment of appropriate play skills

Does the child know how to play appropriately with a variety of toys and objects? Here are some ideas that you can use to assess play skills. You should substitute other activities if you feel these suggestions are not appropriate for your child. Use the summary assessment sheet for appropriate play in Appendix B to record your results.

Suggested assessment activities

- Will the child play appropriately with familiar toys? Put a toy car, soft toy or doll in front of the child and encourage him to play with it. Does he push the car, or pat, cuddle or walk the soft toy or doll? If not, model an appropriate action. Put the child's hand on the car and push it, or put the soft toy or doll in the child's arms and rock it. Now re-administer the task. Does the child play appropriately after practice?

- Will the child use familiar household objects correctly? Put a cup, hat or hairbrush in front of the child and encourage play. Does she use these items appropriately? If not, model appropriate actions, encourage imitation and recheck. Does she use the objects appropriately after practice?
- Will the child look at books, or draw on paper with a pencil or crayon? Put a book in front of the child, or a pencil or crayon and piece of paper. Does he look at the book or use the drawing material appropriately? If not, give some practice and recheck. Does he look at the book or use the drawing material correctly after practice?

If the child did three or four of the tasks on the first attempt, you can move on to the next chapter. If the child is not able to do any of the tasks after practice, then he is probably not yet ready to begin these activities. You should spend more time practising looking together, turn-taking and imitation games. If the child can do one or two of the tasks with or without practice, you should continue to practise appropriate play activities.

Suggestions for practising appropriate play skills

To help a child acquire appropriate play skills, you should follow the same procedures as were suggested earlier for turn-taking and imitation. Model appropriate behaviour and encourage the child to do as you do. Involve the child in the game and continue to play until you are sure she can continue without you. Then you can withdraw and leave her to play independently.

Many of the activities that are appropriate for practising play skills can be introduced when the child is in a group with other children. This issue is discussed in more detail in Chapter 14. In this situation you can involve a few more competent children in the activity so that the child has good models of appropriate play skills, as well as partners for turn-taking. Once these skills are established you can extend the practice activities to other areas of play.

When you begin to help a child develop play skills, it is a good idea to select activities to practise in play contexts that allow for relatively free or unstructured activity, such as in a doll corner, with blocks and model cars or in the sand pit. Children engaged in these types of activities can choose what they want to do. There are few rules about how to play these games. In contrast, activities described as structured include mechanical toys (e.g. a pop-up toy, a wind-up dog), board games (e.g. animal lotto and puzzles) and construction toys (e.g. Duplo). Even bikes, slippery-slides and swings can be described as 'structured' because children are limited in the way they use such materials. Play equipment that can be described as 'structured' is very useful when you are teaching a child more advanced language skills and you need some control over what the child does and says (see Chapters 9 and 10). But in the very early stages of learning to communicate, unstructured materials are more useful because they can be used flexibly, in accord with the child's current interests. Examples of unstructured activities suitable for learning appropriate play activities are shown in Table 6.1.

Table 6.1 Unstructured activities suitable for learning appropriate play activities

Indoors	Outdoors
Games with soft toys and dolls	Sand pit
Tea parties, cooking	Water play
Blocks and cars	Outdoor blocks
Dressing up and pretend games	Informal games without rules

In the types of activities listed in Table 6.1, children are often left to play relatively independently. However, children who have not yet acquired a variety of play skills may need help to begin to use more sophisticated strategies. To help children progress, you will need to organize experiences in these areas to ensure that they are learning appropriate ways of playing with different materials and also hearing appropriate sounds and words. Children who have had difficulty acquiring adequate play skills and speech may not attend to the language they hear. So it is a good idea to encourage the child to both watch and listen as you model new actions and appropriate words during a game (some suggestions are included in the next chapter). This will help the child begin to associate particular words and sounds with the activity.

Remember that to develop appropriate play skills, children need to:

- learn how to explore and manipulate different toys and materials
- hear clear models of appropriate sounds and words during play activities
- engage in games that have a high level of interest
- observe models of appropriate actions that can be imitated and then produced without a model.

You should play the games with the child often (daily if possible). The games can be quite brief (about five minutes). In the early stages when the child is still learning what to do, the child will need to play with the same partner so that the actions and sounds used during the game are consistent. You should comment on what the child is doing using clear, simple words (see Chapter 4 and Appendix F). Try to limit your language to key words. Follow the child's lead as far as possible. Remember that the aim of these games is for the child to learn how to play appropriately with a range of objects and materials.

Taking the next step

Once the child demonstrates appropriate play with a variety of materials, shift your focus from acquisition of appropriate play skills to activities that are accompanied by sounds and early words. This transition is discussed in the next chapter.

Summary

Suggestions are made in this chapter for setting up language acquisition activities with a child who does not yet have the preliminary skills of looking together, turn-taking, imitation and appropriate play. Suggestions are made about ways to assess the child's current skills in each of these areas, and for setting up games and other opportunities for acquiring and practising these skills if necessary.

It is important to remember that children who appear to be more advanced in their development than the level of preliminary skills (level 1) but are having problems in acquiring speech, may, in fact, lack some of the early skills that are described in this chapter. It may seem inappropriate to consider working on these skills with a child who appears to be relatively competent and perhaps has a few recognizable words and phrases, but these skills are the foundations upon which language is based. Children need to have acquired these competences if you are to help with the development of their language.

Finally, it should be noted, again, that although the looking-together skills should precede the other skills discussed in this chapter, there is no fixed order in which the others should be learned. The sequence of 'looking together' followed by 'turn-taking and imitation' and then 'appropriate play' was chosen because it seemed to be a logical progression. In fact, play skills can be taught through turn-taking and imitation. Later, all these skills will be needed when the child learns to talk. They function as tools which are used to acquire other skills, including language, so there is a good reason for helping children to acquire these basic 'tool' skills first. However, the order in which they are introduced should be decided on the basis of the interests and needs of both child and adult.

Chapter 7
Preverbal skills:
programme level 2

Before children begin to produce recognizable words they usually acquire a range of gestures and sounds that they use consistently with particular events or during specific activities. Sometimes the event associated with these gestures and sounds is easily recognized, such as grasping fingers reaching towards the biscuit box for something to eat, or 'tick tick' to look at the watch. Some of the sounds that children make seem like words but have no recognizable meaning although the child appears to use them intentionally to convey a message. For example, Alice uses 'ot' when she wants a special toy and 'bah' when she has wet her nappy. These consistent gestures and sounds or 'words' are sometimes called *performatives* and *protowords*. They are important because they represent a definite level that generally occurs after the child has acquired early turn-taking, imitation and play skills and before a variety of clear words are produced. Their development and use indicates that the child is in the early stages of acquiring effective communication skills (see Chapter 2).

This chapter is primarily concerned with performative sounds because they represent a very useful form of transition for children as they move from crying, babbling and lalling to the production of intelligible speech. If you believe that a child will have difficulty in producing the sounds associated with performatives and, later, speech, you may need to consider the use of manual signs or other forms of alternative or augmented communication as a supplement to speech. This topic is discussed in Chapter 12.

Performatives refer to sounds produced by the child as part of an activity, often involving a game with an adult. 'Boo' is a good example of a performative learned as a key part of the Peek-a-Boo game. Other examples include 'br'mm' which many children learn to vocalize while playing with toy cars, or a sound such as 'whee-ee', used while playing with a model aeroplane. These sounds are initially not used by the child to represent or indicate but are simply part of the routine associated with a particular activity or toy.

Children probably learn performative sounds earlier than words because these sounds are usually easier to say. They are also often produced in an extended or repetitive form, such as 'oo-oo-oo', 'quack quack', 'bang bang'. Such repeated sounds must stand out in the confusion of speech sounds that the child hears. Moreover, they are often associated with physical movements that are related to events that have high interest for the child. 'Bye bye' is a good example here. It is usually paired with a waving movement and is probably produced by children, initially, as a noise paired with an action that is modelled and shaped by an adult at appropriate times. Some examples of common performatives are given in Table 7.1.

Table 7.1 Common performatives

Drop/fall down	'Oh oh'
Food	Lip-smacking noise
Swing	'Whee'
Fire engine	'Ee-or-ee-or'
Bus	'Toot toot'
Dog	'Bow wow'
Aeroplane	'Whoo-oo-oo'
Kiss	Popping lips sound
Favourite blanket	'Er-er'
General excitement	'Yabba-dabba-do' or 'wow'
Waving/going out	'Ta-ta'

No suggestion is made here for assessment of the child's use of proto-words, since it is not appropriate to teach them. It is, however, a good idea to note whether the child is using protowords, because this is further evidence of progress in acquiring language skills. Make a list of any proto-words that you hear and their meaning. This will be useful information for teaching first words (see Chapter 8).

Assessing performative sounds

Check to see if the child is using any performatives and make a list of any sounds that you hear and the situations in which they occur. You may wish to use the summary assessment sheet for performative sounds in Appendix B to record the information that you collect.

Suggested assessment activities

• Will the child produce an appropriate sound as part of a familiar game? If yes, is the sound produced spontaneously or only in imitation? Play 'Peek-a-boo'. Does the child say 'boo' when it is his turn? Play 'Ring-a-Rosie'. Does the child say 'a-tish-oo' or 'down'? If the child does not make any sounds spontaneously, will she do it if you prompt? Repeat each task and model an appropriate sound. Does the child produce the modelled sound?

- Set up a game with model cars, trains, a fire engine or an aeroplane. Does the child make any performative sounds during this game, such as a screeching noise, 'toot' or 'ee-oo-ee-oo' or 'whoo-oo'? Set up a game with a tea-set and doll or soft toy. Does the child make any performative sounds during this activity, such as eating or drinking noises? If the child does not make any sounds spontaneously, will he do it if you prompt? Repeat each task and model an appropriate sound. Does the child produce the modelled sound?
- Set up a game with farm animals. Does the child produce appropriate sounds while playing with the toys, such as 'quack quack', 'baa', 'woof woof' or 'moo'. If the child does not make any sounds spontaneously, will she do it if you prompt? Repeat each task and model an appropriate sound. Does the child produce the modelled sound?

If the child is able to make most of these sounds spontaneously, you will not have to give more practice. If a model is needed, you should provide more opportunities for the child to use these sounds. Remember that children who are already using a few clear words may not like to produce performatives. Some of these children may be ready to move on to the single-word level. You should look for ideas in Chapter 8 to help these children.

Sometimes children begin to produce single words as if they are performatives; for example, 'gone' and 'bye' are often used in this way. These children probably need more practice in producing performative sounds before they move on to the single words. If the child does not make many sounds, you need to provide opportunities to practice some performatives. Children who are having difficulty using consistent and intelligible words to communicate can often be helped to make a start by learning to produce these sounds in association with a familiar activity. Ideas for activities that can be used to introduce a child to performative sounds are set out below. You should model the sounds while taking part in the activity. Once the child is familiar with the sound, encourage imitation. Then watch to find out if the sounds are being used spontaneously during play. Once the child is using some sounds, either alone or with others, you can anticipate the next level by substituting an appropriate word for each sound; for example, 'car' for 'br'mm', 'duck' for 'quack' and so on (see Chapter 8 for more on this process).

Suggestions for practising performative sounds

All the activities listed in Chapter 6 for practising turn-taking, imitation and appropriate play can be used here. Choose activities that can include a sound, such as 'oops' or 'br'mm'. Here are some more ideas.

- Activities associated with soft toys and dolls, tea-sets or blocks and cars and other familiar household objects provide good opportunities for using performative sounds. Some appropriate activities and sounds are shown in Table 7.2.

Table 7.2 Appropriate activities and performative sounds

Doll eat	Smack lips, 'yum yum', 'm'mm'
Pour tea	Continuous 'sh-sh-sh' noise, 'pour-pour'
Teddy drink	Click tongue, 'drink-drink-drink', 'ah'
Teddy sleep	Humming and rocking movement, singing 'la-la-la'
Push car	'Toot', 'br'mm', 'bee-beep', crashing noise
Plane dive	'Whoo-oo-oo'
Blocks fall down	'Oh-oh', 'oops'
Push fire engine	'Ee-oo-ee-oo-ee-oo'
Train go	'Chuff chuff', 'choo choo'

- Model animals have been shown to be a particularly effective means of stimulating performative sounds. Use models of familiar animals that make a sound that the child can imitate. Some appropriate animals and sounds are listed in Table 7.3.

Table 7.3 Appropriate animals and sound

Dog	'Woof woof'
Sheep	'Baa'
Duck	'Quack quack'
Donkey	'Ee-or'
Cat	'Meow'
Pig	'Oink oink'
Turkey	'Gobble gobble'
Cow	'Moo'
Bird	'Tweet tweet'
Horse	'Neigh' or tongue click
Bee or fly	'Bzzz'

- Once the child knows a range of sounds, you should encourage their use during play with other related materials such as animal puzzles and picture books. Appropriate songs can also be taught. These are particularly effective if they can be sung in a group; for example, 'Old Macdonald Had a Farm'. Many children are more likely to produce such sounds if they can hear other children first (see also Chapter 14).
- Some children are interested in the sounds produced by musical instruments. You can introduce a child to these sounds during a game with such instruments. Talk about the sounds that each instrument makes as you play with them, or look at pictures of the instruments (Table 7.4). Once the child is familiar with these sounds, they can be included in action songs such as 'We Can Play on the Big Bass Drum and This Is the Way We Do It'. As with the animal sounds, this type of activity is very effective if played in a group of children who can model appropriate noises and actions for the child.

Table 7.4 Words for sounds made by musical instruments

Drum	'Bang bang'
Bells	'Ding ding'
Horn	'Beep beep'
Trumpet	'Toot toot'
Triangle	'Ting ting'
Tambourine	'Ring ring'

- Use your imagination to find a sound that goes with other familiar objects and events (Table 7.5). Sometimes, at this stage, you can link actions with words by using the words as if they were performatives. For example, saying 'up, up, up' as you climb stairs, saying 'up' as you put your arms up in a game or as you pick a child up from the floor or out of bed. Similarly, you can label actions such as 'walk, walk, walk' as you walk together or make teddy or dolly 'walk'. Other ideas include:
  - 'run, run, run'
  - 'jump, jump, jump'
  - 'down' as the child goes down the slippery slide, or
  - 'in' as you put the blocks away into a box or cupboard.

Table 7.5 Sounds that go with familiar objects and events

Water	'Drip drip', 'woosh'
Flower	'M-mm', 'shiff sniff'
Broom	'Swish swish'
Tree and wind	'Oo-oo'
Smoke	'Sh-sh'
Something sticky/messy	'Ugh', 'yuk'
Going up stairs	'Up, up, up' or 'one, two, three'
Taking off clothes	'Off'
Something good	'Yum yum'
Starting off	'One, two, three, go' or 'ready, set, go'

Even though children are not yet ready to use the full word, they will often be able to produce an approximation, for example:

Adult	**Child**
'up'	'u'
'walk'	'wa, wa'

Games for practising performative sounds

When a child has learned some performative sounds, you should provide a variety of situations where the sounds can be practised. Some useful games include using a 'gone box', a 'surprise bag' or a matching game.

- To play the 'gone box' game, cut an opening in the top of a shoe box, large vegetable box or ice-cream container. Collect 6–8 objects you know the child associates with particular sounds, such as a small clock ('tick tick'), a car ('br'mm'), a cow ('moo') and a toy horn ('toot, toot'). Demonstrate to the child that the object can be posted in the opening after the appropriate sound is made. You will need to keep your hand over the opening, and only allow the child to post the object when the sound has been produced. As you post the object, say 'gone' or 'bye'. Make the game fun. If the child does not make the appropriate sound after a few opportunities, model the task: make the sound and post the object. When all the objects are 'gone', empty the box, reassemble the collection of objects and begin the game again. You can also play this game using pictures instead of objects.

- A similar game can be played with a 'surprise bag'. Hide 6–8 familiar objects in a cloth bag or pillowslip. Let the child feel in the bag for an object and bring it out to show you while making its sound. Once the object has been taken out of the bag, play with it or do an appropriate action, again making a sound; for example:

  car + push + 'br'mm'

  teddy + hug + 'ah'

- Alternatively, you can collect a set of pictures to match the objects and spread them out when you play the game. The child can match each object pulled out of the bag to a picture and make the appropriate sound. The surprise bag and gone box work well together; first the child 'finds' the object in the bag, then 'posts' it in the box after playing with it briefly.

- Other games can be devised to practise performatives. For example, make a tunnel out of cardboard or use a cardboard cylinder. Slide a variety of small objects, such as a car, keys, and comb or farm animals down the tunnel. Make an appropriate sound as the object disappears and reappears again, such as:

  'whee'   'whoo'

  'br'mm'   'boom'

  'oo-oo'   'bang'

  'moo'   'crash'

All these games can be played individually or in a small group. They can also be practised, without the gone box or surprise bag, during daily routines such as snack-time or bath-time. Put a biscuit or piece of fruit in a paper bag and let the child reach in and find it. Pair a sound with the food as it appears, such as 'm-mm' and 'yum yum'. Or 'hide' a floating object under the water and make a noise as you release it. A ping-pong ball works well in this game. The surprise game with its objects is a useful activity to take on car outings and to appointments with the doctor. It will help to keep the child occupied.

Daily activities

It is a good idea to set yourself the aim of trying to use a sound or word to accompany your own and the child's actions as you play together or carry out daily activities. Some examples include:

- 'out' as you go out the door
- 'oh oh' when you drop an object or stumble
- 'on' as you put on socks and shoes
- 'wash, wash, wash' and 'rub, rub, rub' as you wash and dry face and hands before a snack
- 'whee' as you spin the child around.

This way you will be constantly providing models for the child to imitate while reinforcing the idea that sounds go with actions.

Taking the next step

When the child has acquired some performatives, you can begin to pair a single word with these sounds to encourage the child to replace the sounds with appropriate words. Once children begin to use performatives spontaneously, you will find that they gradually substitute words for the sounds without any extra help. Now it is time to move to the next level in the language programme. The next chapter provides an outline of procedures to use for helping a child begin to use single words.

Summary

Ideas for assessment and practise of performative sounds are introduced in this chapter. This level in the language programme is an important intermediate stage for a child who has the preliminary skills described in Chapter 6 but is not ready to produce recognizable words. Over time, most children begin to substitute words for performative sounds and protowords. Experience with children who are having difficulty in acquiring speech skills suggests that learning to produce performatives can provide a very useful bridge between meaningless babble and first words.

Chapter 8
First words: programme level 3

Children's first communicative acts are usually related to real events that have a high level of interest for them, such as Daddy's car, a passing aeroplane, or the family pet. Later, the child learns to use gestures, sounds and words to make things happen or to obtain desired objectives, such as food, drink or comfort. This chapter is concerned with children's language development at the point where they begin to utter their first words. It begins with suggestions for assessing the current communication skills of children who are starting to produce intelligible single words. Specific words that are likely to be acquired by children at this stage of development are identified, together with ideas for games and other activities that may provide opportunities for practising these words.

As discussed in Chapter 2, detailed studies of children who are just beginning to talk have shown that, initially, they use words to:

- indicate the existence of something that interests them (for example, 'look', 'there')
- obtain objects and services that they want (for example, a toy, food or help to climb on to a swing)
- regulate other people's actions. This may include *protest* (for example, 'don't do that'; 'no'.) or a *request for attention or service* (for example, 'watch me'; 'come and play'; 'wash hands').

Once children begin to communicate these types of meanings intentionally with others using a few consistent gestures and sounds, opportunities can be provided to help them learn some useful words to use during such communication. This learning process can take place in a variety of different situations during the day. However, before introducing games to stimulate early speech, you will need to find out what gestures, sounds and words a child is already using to communicate. The best way to do this is through unstructured observation. For example, you may decide to observe the child carefully during daily routines or ask a parent or carer what meanings the child is expressing and how these are expressed. Alternatively, you can take a sample of the child's language. You can also assess the child's production and imitation of single words by using a structured activity. These different methods of assessment are described below. Suggestions are then made for selecting new words to practise. Issues associated with the emergence of the communicative intentions identified above are explored more fully in Chapter 10.

Choice of language for children whose home language is not English

Many children belong to families where the language used in the home is not English, though English is the main language used outside the home; at the shops, the school, the church and so on. As these children begin to talk, their parents are sometimes uncertain about which language the children should be learning; the 'home' language or that of the dominant group in the community. Children are very adaptable and once they begin to use one language, they are usually able to recognize contexts where 'other' words should be used. For example, they learn to say 'num' at home and 'drink' at preschool, or 'shi-shi' at home and 'wee' at school. If you are the child's main carer, you should probably begin by helping the child to learn the language you like to use at home. If you are working with the child outside the home, then you may not know the child's home language and so have no choice about which language to use in your practice games. However, it may be a good idea to talk to the child's family to identify some words from home that you can include in your programme. This issue is discussed in some detail in Chapter 13.

Suggested assessment activities

Children's communication skills can be assessed in a variety of ways that can be described as 'unstructured' or 'structured'. An unstructured assessment technique means that the methods you use are quite informal and flexible, mainly involving careful observation of communication in everyday contexts. A structured assessment is more formal, meaning that the procedures are implemented using fairly specific guidelines. Both these approaches will give you useful information. You may decide to begin with an unstructured assessment technique, such as a language sample and supplement the information by using a structured assessment procedure. Examples of both unstructured and structured procedures for assessing children's communicative behaviour are described below.

Unstructured assessment of first words

Make a list of the meanings the child is able to express through gestures, consistent sounds or recognizable words. This information can be collected in three ways:

- *Observation*: Over a period of several days, make a list of all the gestures, sounds and words that you observe the child using. Also note the meaning of each item. If this is not obvious, follow the clues you use to recognize whether the child is expressing some communicative intent, such as any actions that occur, or the activity in which the gestures, sounds or words are used. It is sometimes helpful to record whether the item is used spontaneously or in imitation, what is going on at the time, who the child is talking to and what you think he or she is trying to say. You may wish to record the information using the observation record form for single words in Appendix C.
- *Parent report*: Ask a parent or carer to make a list of the gestures, sounds and words they know the child uses. They should also describe how and in what contexts these meanings are expressed. You may wish to give them a copy of the observation record form for sounds, gestures, words or phrases (in Appendix C) for recording this information.
- *Language sample*: Set up an activity the child likes, such as a game with teddy or looking at a book. Play the game with the child for 5–10 minutes. Keep a note pad and pen beside you and list all the child's communicative acts (gestures, sounds and words). A tape or video-recorder is useful here, because it allows you to concentrate on interacting with the child during the activity. You can check later for any instances of communicative behaviour. Again, you should note any contextual clues that will help you understand the child's meaning. Guidelines for taking a language sample are provided in Appendix A.

Having collected a list of the ways in which the child is currently communicating, you can sort them into one of the five broad types of meaning:

- people: names: Mum, Daddy, sibling names, family pets
- object: labels: real things ('ball', 'car')
- actions: related to movement ('look', 'fall down')
- modifiers: related to conditions and states ('more', 'hot', 'blue', 'in')
- other words: items that you are unsure how to classify, including socially useful words ('bye', 'no').

You should also note how each meaning is expressed. Is it by:

- gestures (G): pointing
- sounds (S):   'br'mm'
- words (W):   'ba' (ball)?

Some examples of two children's communication lists are shown in Table 8.1.

Table 8.1 Children's communication lists

Names	Objects	Actions	Modifiers	Other
Johan's word list (4 years, 3 months)				
Bubba (W)	car (S)	go (W)	wet (W)	gone (G)
Dada (W)	hat (W)	hide (G)	hot (W)	no (W)
Mummy (W)		fall down(W)	more (G)	ta (W)
Spot (W)		come (G)		there (G)
Ya Ya (Teddy:W)		look (G)		
		out (G)		
Laaya's word list (3 years, 9 months)				
Ibu (Mum:W)	book (G)	shi-shi (W)	hot (S)	kai-kai (W)
Ayah (Dad:W)	(ba)nana (W)	eat (G)	smelly(S)	ta (W)
	plane (S)	go up (G)	in (G)	oops (W)
	car (S)	open (G)		

If you are unsure how to classify a particular item, put it where it seems most appropriate to you. This is your list, and you should sort the words in a way that makes sense to you. (The list of first words in Appendix D may be useful here.) This information will give you a good record of the way the child is communicating, whether words are used only to obtain objects and never to protest or attract attention, and whom the child talks to most often, such as Granny or a helper at the crèche. This information will be very useful when you are deciding which objectives to select for helping the child to learn some single words.

Structured assessment of first words

As an alternative to the informal methods described above, a child's current communication skills can be assessed by using an activity that the child enjoys, such as a tea party or a car game. While playing the game, you will need to ensure that the child has opportunities to use appropriate words, spontaneously or in imitation. This information will supplement the list of words and meanings you have collected from parental reports and your own observations. Moreover, since the strategies you will use to practise new language skills include imitation of an adult speech model, this assessment procedure will help you find out if the child can imitate a word that has just been heard. Note that some children are more interested in activities than in objects, and for these children, action words (for example, 'go', 'jump', 'fall down') rather than object labels are often learned first.

When working through the assessment activities described below, it is important to allow the child time to respond to each task. Young children often need more time to reply to requests to 'do' or 'say' than might be expected for older children, so try to wait for the child to attempt to do what you have asked.

Spontaneous speech

• Will the child label a familiar object or action as part of a surprise bag game? Use the surprise bag described in Chapter 7. Find a cloth bag, a pillowslip or a large paper bag. Collect four objects that are familiar to the child. Label the items and let the child watch as you put each item into the bag. Now let the child feel in the bag for one of the objects. As the child takes it out, say 'What is it?', or 'What have you found?'. If the child begins to play with the item, say 'What are you doing' or 'What is (child's name) doing?' Can the child tell you? If he or she cannot label the object or use a word to describe what the object is doing (e.g. '[car] go'), look at the item carefully and ask again, 'What is it?' Repeat with the other objects. Keep a list of any words the child says. Your aim, here, is to find out if the child can label four familiar objects or actions. Some appropriate objects to use in a surprise bag and words to use with them are listed in Table 8.2.

Table 8.2 The surprise bag: objects and words

Ball	'Gone'
Car	'Go'
Key	'In'
Cup	'Drink'
Spoon	'More', 'eat'
Fruit	'Banana', 'apple'
Shoe	'On'
Doll	'Baby'
Book	'Open', 'read'
Hat	'Off'
Brush	'Brush'
Duck	'Quack'

Use any other objects that you know interest the child. Does the child label three or four of the objects?

• Will the child label a familiar object or action in a picture book? Find a set of pictures or a picture book that includes objects or people that are familiar to the child. Sit beside the child and look at the pictures. Ask 'What's that?', 'Who is that?' or 'What is (child's name) doing?'. Keep a list of any words the child says. Does the child say an appropriate word for three or four of the pictures?

Imitated speech

• Will the child imitate a model of an appropriate word during an activity with an adult? Repeat the surprise bag game described above, but this time use four objects or pictures of objects that you think the child might recognize but cannot already label. As the child takes each item out of the bag, ask 'What is it?' or 'What is happening?'. If the child cannot reply, model an appropriate word. Say 'It's a . . . ' or 'She's . . . ing'. Then encourage the child to repeat the word. Say 'You say . . . '. Remember that your aim here is to find out if the child can imitate your words. Keep a list of any words the child imitates. You may find the summary assessment sheet for level 4, early sentences (Appendix B) useful here. For this activity, you should select object labels and action words that are relatively easy for the child to say. For English-speaking children, some suitable words are listed in Table 8.3.

Table 8.3 Easy object and action words

Bath	Duck	Mat	Pig
Bell	Dog	Mop	Pompom
Bird	(Fall) down		Pull
	Eat		

You could include any other objects that may interest the child. Try to select items that have only one syllable and begin with a consonant such as 'b', 'm', 'p', 'd' or vowel sounds such as 'e' or 'a' that you know the child can say. Keep a record of what the child says. Does the child imitate at least four words appropriately?

• Will the child imitate a model of an appropriate word while looking at a book with an adult? Find a set of four pictures or a picture book that includes objects and activities that the child cannot already label. Repeat the procedure that was described in the previous activity. Try to elicit an appropriate word and if the child cannot say the word, model it and encourage imitation. Does the child imitate at least four words appropriately?

If the child is able to label at least two of the items spontaneously or in imitation, he or she has appropriate skills to take part in the language activities described in this chapter. If the child is unwilling or unable to say the words or imitate your model, you may need to go back to the imitation and turn-taking section in Chapter 6 (programme level 1), and encourage further use of performatives (Chapter 7: programme level 2).

Suggestions for practising first words

Once you have pinpointed precisely the meanings that the child is communicating and how this is done, you can begin to develop ideas for new words to practise. Look at the list of words, gestures and sounds that you compiled during the assessment activities you have just carried out. If most of the list comprises gestures, you should look at the previous chapter, which outlines ways of helping the child to produce performative sounds. Such sounds are often a useful bridge for the child who has acquired a range of gestures to express meaning but who does not use many clear words. If the child has a rich collection of gestures and is communicating quite complex meaning through them, but lacks intelligible words, you should consider including some signs among the ideas you are developing for practice activities. Indeed, when working with any child who is experiencing difficulties in learning to talk it can be helpful to pair either a gesture or natural sign with a new word that is being practised. Such signs and gestures provide a visual prop for the child and facilitate, rather than interfere with, the process of learning to use intelligible words. The use of signs and gestures to supplement speech is discussed in Chapter 12.

The strategy suggested to help a child begin to produce new words is derived from skills acquired during turn-taking and imitation games. In these games, the child learned to watch and copy actions and sounds. It is also based on the strategy used by carers when they ask a question and then answer it themselves, knowing that the infant does not yet have the skills to reply (see Chapter 4 and Appendix F). Examples might include the sequences: 'what shall we do now? Have a bath!' and 'Where's your bottle? There!'. Children who have problems learning to talk need to hear clear models of new words, and to have opportunities to practise these words.

The child needs to be reminded of an appropriate word to use in a particular situation, hear a model of the word that can be copied and then use the word without a model, soon after it has been practised and before it is forgotten. This has been called the *'conversation-imitation-conversation'* or C-I-C strategy (Horstmeier and MacDonald, 1978). The C-I-C strategy has three parts:

- conversation (C1)
- imitation (I)
- conversation (C2).

Some examples of the C-I-C strategy in use

Jara is washing teddy in 'home corner'

C1	Adult:	'Jara, what's happening?'
Jara:	no reply	
I	Adult:	'Jara, say (or tell me) "wash"'
Jara:	'Wash'	
C2	Adult:	'Jara, what's happening?'
Jara:	'Wash'	

Ben wants something to eat

C1	Adult:	'Ben, what do you want?'
Ben:	no reply	

I	Adult:	'Ben, say (or tell me) "bickie"'
Ben:	'Bickie'	
C2	Adult:	'What do you want?'
Ben:	'Bickie'	

Shauna is trying to show her mother something interesting

C1	Mother:	'What can you see?'
Shauna:	no reply	
I	Mother:	'Shauna, say (or tell me) "balloon"'
Shauna:	'Balloon'	
C2	Mother:	'What can you see?'
Shauna:	'Balloon'	

In these sequences, the adult first gives the child an opportunity to produce an appropriate word correctly. If the child cannot do this, the adult models an appropriate word and encourages imitation. When the child imitates the word, the adult repeats the original question, giving the child an opportunity to use the word without a model.

It is very important to remember that you should never ask a child to say or imitate a word more than three times. Always avoid confrontation. If the child does not respond to the imitation request after three tries, leave this word and try again another time. If the child refuses to attempt the word over a number of days, then drop it and find another word to practise or go back to an earlier level in the language programme, such as imitation of performative sounds (Chapter 7).

Selecting new words for practice

To help a child learn new words, first identify which words will be useful for the child. You can begin with four or five words and expand the list to as many as ten words once the child has learned the rules of the new language game.

Next, you need to select an enjoyable activity or routine which provides opportunities for you and the child to use the selected words, such as during games with teddy or a doll, during a ride in the car, at snack-time or bath-time. Finally, you can begin to use the C-I-C strategy to help the child learn to use the words appropriately. You may find it a little difficult to use this technique at first, but you will be surprised how quickly it will become a natural part of your interaction with the child. Examples of words that might be suitable to include in a list for a child at the single-word level are included in the list of first words in Appendix D.

Children need to acquire a variety of words from the five categories listed earlier, including names of people, object labels, actions, modifiers and other words. At first, they will mainly need words to label objects and familiar people, a few action words and some modifiers. Socially useful words, such as 'bye' and 'ta', also need to be acquired, but these are usually learned during the child's daily activities and, as a result, do not need to be deliberately targeted. However, some children do not acquire these words naturally and need some help.

Finally, it is worth noting that politeness words such as 'please' and 'ta' should not be introduced until the child has begun to use a number of different words to communicate. These words often seem important to adults, but they can cause difficulties for the child with poor communication skills. Both child and carer can become very frustrated when the child replies to a question such as 'tell me what you want' by saying 'please' or 'ta'. In this situation, the child thinks that the desired answer has been given, whereas the adult still does not have a satisfactory answer to the original question. For example:

Child: 'Ta' (pointing at the cupboard)
Adult: 'What do you want?'
Child: 'Ta' (still pointing at cupboard)
Adult: 'Tell me what you want'
Child: 'Ta'
Adult: 'I don't know what you want'.
Child: 'Ta'.

It is a good idea to wait until the child has acquired the words needed to express basic needs and interests before you begin to encourage these socially useful words.

Which words should you choose to teach first?

Most children begin to talk using labels for things that interest them very much. For example, apart from 'Mum' and 'Dad', many children say 'ball', 'bus' or 'car' first. Look at the list you have made of the child's gestures, sounds and words. It is a good idea to start with these. If the child is using a gesture or sound to communicate a specific meaning, choose an appropriate word for this meaning and put it on your list of words to teach. This list may include words for objects that are important for the child, for familiar people, actions or modifier words. Make a list of up to 10 target words, including a few that the child already knows as 'success' items. Now decide how to practise the words. Some can be taught during daily routines. For example, 'out' can be practised when it is time to go outside, 'come' or 'look' when the child tugs at an adult's clothing and indicates need for help or attention. Other words such as 'car', 'ball', 'baby', 'sit', 'go', 'pat', 'up', 'in' and 'out' can be taught in a game or during daily routines.

Suggestions for practising new words

Having decided which words you will try to teach the child, choose a game or daily activity where the words can be used. Some ideas for appropriate games or activities are listed below. If you decide to carry out your practice as part of a game, then you will need to make a list of the target words and collect any materials required. You may decide to monitor what happens during the game by keeping running records of target words used by the child, using a small notebook, sticky notes or a data-collection sheet such as the observation record form for single words included in Appendix C.

One of the most effective contexts for practising new words occurs within the events and activities that occur spontaneously during the day. For teaching in these settings, it is helpful to have a list of your target words displayed in a place where everyone who has contact with the child can see it. For example, put the list on the refrigerator or family notice-board at home, or on daily programme sheets or the notice board at preschool or at the daycare centre. A regular babysitter or nanny can also be given a copy of the list.

To practise the language goals you have selected, look for appropriate situations during the day, or set up an activity with the materials you have decided to use. Play with the materials while you follow the child's gaze and, at an appropriate time, introduce a C-I-C sequence using one of your target words. To practise a word you should first give the child an opportunity to hear it used in association with the object, action or event. For example, before attempting to teach 'Mum', find a photograph of her and ask 'Where's Mum' or 'Show me Mum'. If the child demonstrates comprehension of the word 'Mum', then you can begin to introduce the C-I-C strategy:

C1	Adult:	'Who's that?' (pointing to picture of Mum)
Child:	no reply	
I	Adult:	Say (or tell me) 'Mum'
Child:	'Mum'	
C2	Adult:	'Who is it?'
Child	'Mum.'	

Keep a check on what the child says for each item on your list. Once a correct word (or approximation for the word) is produced in the C1 condition over a few days, you can probably drop that item from your list and select another word to teach. Now tell everyone who has contact with the child that she can say 'Mum', and encourage them to give her opportunities for her to use the word. Giving plenty of opportunities for the child to use the word throughout the day, with different partners, helps the child both to remember the word and to practise using it. These opportunities ensure that newly acquired language skills are generalized to new contexts, outside the practice situations you are providing. The words you decide to teach should have meanings that are important to the child, and be useful during daily events and with different partners. This will help to ensure that the child continues to use the words and does not forget them. There will then be less need for you to check, later, that the child has not forgotten the words and is still using them both spontaneously and appropriately.

Finally, try to remember that you should always follow the child's lead. Embed your practice in games and activities that he is interested in and enjoys. Encourage the child to respond and always allow enough time. Ask only three times. Avoid confrontation.

Activities to use when teaching a child to use new words

Names of family members, pets or friends

Check your list of the child's gestures, sounds and words. Are there three or four items for family names or the names of pets (if any) or friends? If not, here are some suggestions for ways to encourage the use of these words, using the C-I-C strategy:

* Play a game such as 'Here We Go Round the Mulberry Bush' with family members, friends or other children. Let each person call out in turn the name of the next person to model an action for the group to copy.
* Use model people from Lego or a doll's house. Play with the models, label them using the names on your list.
* Use two-dimensional figures such as cutout pictures of people. Follow the procedure described above.
* Draw faces on your fingertips. Say 'Where's Daddy?' Hide a finger and 'find' it again. Repeat with other names.
* Collect pictures and photographs from home. Put them in an album. Look at the pictures and label them. 'There's Winnie' (family pet). 'Here's (child's name)'.
* Cut pictures from magazines with the child and label them appropriately; 'Mummy', 'Daddy', 'Granny', 'Uncle', 'Peter', 'Baby'.

Note that the ideas listed above move from the three-dimensional and concrete to increasingly two-dimensional and abstract.

Names of familiar objects (such as ball, hat, car)

Check your list of the child's gestures, sounds and words for object labels. Are there 8–10 names of familiar objects? If not, you will need to find opportunities to practise such words.

When you begin to practise word labels, first check that the child knows the meaning of the words you plan to teach. Before playing a game, ask the child to show you, give you, or touch the items as you label them. If the child is not sure of the meaning of the words, you will need to allow plenty of opportunities to associate the sound of words with the objects they represent. Follow the steps outlined earlier for teaching family names.

Suggestions for activities to use

- Use real objects that interest the child. Put them in a surprise bag. Take turns to take out one object at a time and encourage the child to label the object as it is taken out.
- Collect a set of pictures to match the real objects you are teaching. Let the child match object to picture and label it at the same time.
- Make a gone box (see Chapter 7). Allow the child to 'post' an object only when it has been labelled.
- Find a simple picture lotto that uses familiar objects. Have the child name the picture before matching it on the board. This is a useful game to play with a small group who will provide good language models for the child.
- Looking at a book provides a good opportunity for talking. Collect the pictures you have used in the activities described above and mount them in a photo album or use clear plastic covers that can be clipped together to make a book. The child should label the picture before turning a page.

When selecting labels to teach a child, remember two points:

- Find words for objects and events that are relevant and interesting for the child. Look at the world from the child's point of view and select words that the child will find useful. Remember, objects that move, make a noise and are colourful are most likely to interest children. A sample list of words that could be used is included in the list of first words in Appendix D.
- Select words that the child will not find too difficult to say. Listen to the sounds the child is already making and select words that include these sounds. You should note, however, that children who can make a particular sound during vocal play (such as 'f-f-f') might not be able to make the sound intentionally. So listen carefully before you select a word to teach. A list of the order in which most children acquire consonants is listed in the articulation development norms in Appendix E. Suggestions for ways to describe how particular sounds are made are included in Chapter 11.

Words for actions (such as go, put, give)

Check your list of the child's words. Are there at least 10 words for actions? If not, you will need to give some practice in using action words.

Action words are important because the child needs these to make simple sentences. However, these words lack a clear physical referent. For example, you cannot pick up, hide, put or hold 'walk'. As a result, such words are often difficult to learn. Many children who have begun to use a number of object labels are very slow to use words for actions. If a child has 30–40 object labels it is time to learn some action words as well. One way to begin to teach these words is to pair a word to a gesture already used by the child to communicate an action meaning. For example, many children express 'come', 'want', 'look', 'out(side)', 'all gone' in their gestures and body language long before they use a word. Use the C-I-C strategy to help the child begin to add words to these gestures and actions. Use daily routines such as bath-time or snack-times, or set up a game that will involve activities appropriate for the words you want to practise. Structure the activity so that the child has to name an action before doing it, or as you do it.

Suggestions for activities to use

• Have a tea party with teddy or a doll, or play with blocks and cars. Label the actions as you play: 'go', 'stop', 'crash', 'bang', 'sleep', 'walk', 'jump'. Use these procedures during snack-time, labelling what you are doing as in 'eat', 'drink', 'more'. Label what is happening when washing hands; 'wash', 'rub', '(tap) off'.
• Play with dough or clay. As you manipulate it, label the actions: 'pat', 'roll', 'squash', 'poke', 'press', 'pull', 'pinch'.
• Look at a book with pictures of adults and children involved in different activities. Label the action component of the pictures as you look at the book; such as 'sleep', 'eat', 'wash', 'run', 'jump', 'push', 'cut'.
• Play 'Follow the Leader'. Let a small group of children play with you, each child taking turns to name an action. Or use the same procedure to play 'Here We Go Round the Mulberry Bush'.
• Play charades with a small group. One person can mime an action and the other children guess the action being mimed.

During all the activities described above, remember to ask what the child is doing or what she wants you to do. Using the C-I-C strategy, you can teach words such as

tea party, snack-time:	put, pour, drink, eat, all gone
play dough:	cut, roll, poke, squash, put
model cars, animals:	go, stop, walk, run, push, ride, get
soft toys or dolls:	sleep, wash, walk, jump, fall down

Once the child is able to use a few clear action words appropriately, without having just heard a model as in C2 in the C-I-C strategy, use a binary-choice question to provide some help in producing correct words. Ask 'Do you want to cut or paste?' or 'Do you want to build or climb?'. This will help the child who is not quite ready, to answer such questions spontaneously, without a prompt.

Binary choice is a useful strategy to use in many different situations throughout the day. Use it when you are asking the child what he wants at times involving, for example:

food:	'peanut butter or honey?'
service:	'Mummy pick you up or get your blanket?'
play:	'blocks or puzzles?'.

Remember to reinforce the child's choice in your response, as in 'You want . . . ?' or 'Shall we have . . . ?'. This strategy is best introduced when the child can see the objects or activities they can choose from. Use real objects and pictures to get started. You can drop these prompts later.

Modifiers (such as hot, wet, more, big)

Modifier words can be taught in games and activities such as those described above. Children will need plenty of opportunities to hear these words in association with the condition they represent before they will begin to use them. Most children learn some modifiers early; words such as 'wet', 'hot', 'more', 'big'. Others are learned only after the child has a variety of words for entities and actions. Some suitable words to teach include:

prepositions:	in, on, under, up, down
adjectives:	little, my, more, yummy, yuckie
colour names:	red, blue, yellow

Socially useful words (such as bye, ta)

Words that can be described as 'socially useful' are usually learned during appropriate daily activities. Many children learn 'bye' first. As noted earlier, some children have a problem in communicating their ideas and needs to another person if they have already learned to use words such as 'ta' or 'thank you'. These 'polite' words convey no information and if the child is able to use only one or two words at a time, words such as 'please' and 'thank you' take the place of other words that convey more of the child's meaning. It is better to keep such polite phrases for a later stage, when the child is able to use them in addition to the words that carry useful information. However, you should encourage the child to say 'hi' or 'hello' and 'bye' (initially easier to say than 'goodbye'), because these words help the child to interact successfully with other people. Another useful word is 'goodnight' or 'ni-ni'.

Signs as a supplement to speech

Most children, including those with low muscle tone or a motor disability, can be helped to learn words, particularly high-interest words, if the child's communication partner pairs a consistent gesture or sign with the word. Children often begin to communicate their needs by using a gesture, such as pointing to indicate an object of interest, or an action to convey some other meaning. Once they learn to talk, these gestures and actions are replaced by words. In the same way, adults often pair words that have no physical referent with a gesture, as in 'look' plus pointing at the object of interest, 'come' plus a beckoning movement, 'stop' plus positioning the hand upright and 'sit' plus pointing downwards. These gestures provide a visual or tactile prop that aids comprehension of the speaker's meaning. In addition, the visual cue helps the child in the early levels of language acquisition to associate a particular pattern of speech sounds with a specific referent. If you are helping a child who is at this level you should consider encouraging the use of gestures or signs as a bridge to first words.

Pairing a gesture or sign with a word is one strategy that may help your child to learn labels for objects that cannot always be physically present, such as 'toilet', 'car', 'plane', or actions like 'wash', 'sleep', 'dig', 'gone', and other meanings such as 'more', 'little', 'under'. The child may first learn to use a gesture or sign rather than a word, but these are dropped once the child can produce the word intelligibly. The use of gestures and signs as an aid to communication prior to the acquisition of intelligible speech can be particularly useful for children who are not yet physically able to make a variety of speech sounds. See Chapter 12 for a more detailed discussion of the use of gestures and signs in early communication.

Learning to use words effectively

Earlier in this chapter it was suggested that children usually begin to use words first to indicate the existence of something that interests them very much, such as an aeroplane overhead or a butterfly in the garden. Later, they use words to obtain objects, such as a new toy, food or a drink and to regulate and control other people's actions by protesting, as in 'stop, don't do that' or requesting attention or services from an adult, with 'look at me' or 'help me climb here'.

In the early stages of a language programme, the primary goal is to increase the number of different words that the child uses. However, it is also important to check that the child is using words in different ways, not just to label objects or people. If you are concerned about the way in which a child is using language, read Chapter 10 on communicative intentions. In that chapter, procedures are described to help ensure that a child who is only just beginning to talk learns to use language in a variety of ways.

Whatever words you select to practise, here are some important points to remember:

- Follow the child's lead. Try to implement your objectives in activities that engage the child's interest.
- Make sure the child understands what is expected of her during the activity or game. She needs to know how the game is played.
- Make sure the child associates a new word with appropriate objects or activities before you expect to hear the word being used, whether in imitation or spontaneously. Provide plenty of opportunities for him to hear the word used in conjunction with the object or activity.
- In choosing words to practise, always include a few words that the child already knows. This helps to ensure a feeling of success.
- Do not expect the child to learn all the items on your list at one time. It may take several sessions before a child will attempt a new word and only two or three words will be learned at a time.
- Give plenty of opportunities for the new words to be practised.
- Accept any attempt by the child to say a new word. Words should gradually become more intelligible.
- Use naturally occurring situations as much as possible to introduce and practise new words. This will help ensure that the words are meaningful to the child. Special times are sometimes used to give extra opportunity to practise new words, but most language learning will take place in natural contexts.
- Tell everyone who has regular contact with the child about the words that you are practising. Parents, siblings, grandparents, the babysitter, preschool teacher and other familiar adults should be aware of your language objectives.
- Keep practice sessions short. Do not expect the child to continue participating in an activity when bored or tired. Several short productive sessions are far more effective than one long one.
- If a child does not attempt to use a word after you have modelled it and encouraged imitation over several days, you may need to drop that item from your list and chose another word to teach.
- Make sure that the child has plenty of opportunities to practise new words during routine daily activities. Sometimes, this is the only way teach new words. Some suitable times are:
  - at meal and snack-times: ask the child to say 'more', 'eat' or 'juice' before you offer something to eat or drink
  - in the bathroom: ask the child to say 'on' or 'wash' before turning on the tap or washing hands, 'soap' before taking the soap
  - during dressing and undressing: ask the child to label items of clothing as they are put on or taken off. Say 'up', 'off' as pants and socks are pulled on and off.

Taking the next step

Children who have been slow to talk often prefer to communicate using single words only, or, in some instances, phrases associated with daily routines or rituals, such as 'there yare', 'cuppa tea' and 'ready-set-go'. So it is important that, once the child is using a variety of types of words in different situations, you should move on to the next levels in the language programme (levels 4 and 5 in Chapter 9). These are concerned with helping the child combine single words into phrases, sentences and longer utterances. The use of the morphemes of English is also considered.

Summary

For most children and their families, first words represent a major developmental milestone. These words are usually derived from aspects of their experience that are highly salient and they want to communicate about with others. In this chapter, suggestions are made about ways of assessing the current skills of a child who appears to be at the point of uttering first words. Ideas for words that children often produce at this stage of their development are identified and suggestions made about games and activities within which these words can be acquired. Once children are producing a variety of single words and beginning to combine them into two-word utterances, it is time to move on to the next chapter, which examines children's early word combinations and sentences.

Chapter 9
Early sentences and extending meaning: programme levels 4 and 5

Once the child has 10–20 words for people and objects, and 5–10 action or other types of words, you may begin to hear these words being combined into simple sentences such as 'ball gone' or ' boy there'. These early sentences reflect the way the child sees the objects and events. They usually involve identification of an object of interest, plus a comment about the object ('bird gone', 'dolly eat', 'truck there') or the addition of a word that refers to something or someone associated with that object ('Daddy spoon', 'more bickie', 'go car'). This chapter is concerned with these early word combinations and sentences. Suggestions are made about assessing these skills and ways of encouraging further development.

In the second part of the chapter, suggestions are made about one other useful aspect of language: morphology, or the way that the meaning of words is extended to show, for example, tense, mood and number. It should be noted that this part of the chapter is specific to morphemes of the English language.

Programme level 4

Combining words into sentences: early sentences

Research has shown that when children begin to combine words, they are expressing their understanding of relationships they perceive to exist between entities (people and objects) in their environment. In combining words into simple phrases and sentences, they appear to follow common rules. For example, a child who uses 'Mum' and 'up', might at first combine them into 'Mum up' to ask to be picked up, then say 'Mum pick up' and later 'Mum, pick me up'. The order in which the words are combined reflects the child's perception of the relationship between the items or events that have been labelled. In the case of the statement 'Mum up', the child first labelled 'Mum' as the agent (person or actor) involved and then labelled 'up' as the action or event that was of interest.

Children usually begin to combine words by using labelling words or nouns that represent people or objects with action words or verbs that represent the 'action' in an event; what is done by a person or to an object. Examples of word labels include 'doll', 'hat', 'car' or 'Mummy', while action words that might be used with these labels include 'wash', 'put', 'go' and 'give'. Words to indicate location might then be added, such as 'there', 'under' and possibly some modifiers for the labelling words such as 'big', 'hot' and 'blue' or introducer (socially useful) words such as 'bye'. Other examples of these categories of words are set out in the list of first words (Appendix D). The listener often has to consider the situation or context in which the word combination is spoken in order to know what the child means. For example 'Dad car' could mean 'Dad's car', 'Dad drives the car' or 'Dad is in the car'. Knowing the context is crucial for understanding the meaning of children's early sentences.

There are 10 rules that children usually follow when they begin to string words together. These rules tend to be acquired in the same order by most children, regardless of the language spoken in the child's environment. The rules are listed in Table 9.1.

Table 9.1 10 early rules of word combination

Rule	Example
Agent + action	Mum go
Action + object	Push car
Agent + object	Mummy (gives) bickie
Modifier (possession) + object label	Daddy car, my doll
Modifier (recurrence) + object label	More bickie
Modifier (attribution) + object label	Big car
Agent/object + location	Car there
Action + location	Fall down
Negation + any word	No want, no bickie
Introducer + any word	Bye Mum, see train

Once children have begun to use a variety of single words, they usually start to string words together spontaneously. However, experience has shown that children who are slow in using first words are also slow to use simple phrases and sentences (Paul and Fountain, 1999). This chapter provides guidelines for helping children move from a single-word level to the production of two- and three-word phrases and sentences. As in the preceding chapters, suggestions are made for assessing the child's current language skills using both unstructured observation and structured games. Strategies are then described that can be used to help children begin to combine their words and thus move to a higher level in the language development sequence.

Suggested assessment activities

You will need to begin by checking if the child is combining words. You can do this using either informal observation or more formal methods of assessment, as set out below. You may decide to use the summary assessment sheet for level 4, early sentences (Appendix B) to record your information about the child's word combinations.

Unstructured observation of two-or-more word combinations

Three procedures – parent report, systematic observation and language sampling – can be used to assess a child who appears to be ready to combine words into sentences. These techniques were also suggested in the previous chapter for assessing the child at the single-word level. However, this time you will be looking for evidence of the rules that the child is expressing, rather than for a list of the words that are used.

- *Parent report:* Ask a parent or carer to make a list of any utterances that the child produces that include two words or more. Request that, if possible, the list include at least 20 phrases or sentences. You may decide to suggest that the observer use the observation record form that is included in Appendix C for utterances of two, three or more words. The information recorded on this form will help you recognize the meaning that the child wants to convey. You can also classify each utterance listed in terms of the rule that is expressed. For example, Table 9.2 shows a list that was collected by Jane's mother. Her teacher classified each two-word utterance in terms of the 10 rules listed earlier in Table 9.1.

Table 9.2 Jane's list of two-word phrases

Utterance	Rule
'Daddy car'	agent + object
'Go car'	action + object
'Blue car'	modifier + object
'Me go'	agent + action
'Me there'	agent + location
'Go down'	action + location
'Me down	agent + location

- *Systematic observation:* During normal activities with the child, record any utterances of two words or more that you hear, using the observation record form in Appendix C. When you have collected about 20 utterances you can classify them in terms of the rules that are being expressed.
- *Language sampling:* Your aim, here, is to collect a representative sample of the child's speech by making a tape- or video-recording of a 5–10-minute play session. You can then replay the tape or video segment and record exactly what the child did and said. Before you begin,

you will need to choose two different sets of material for the child to play with during the session. For younger children, suitable materials might include a tea-set and doll or soft toy, farm animals and a barn, model cars with a box for a garage, and several picture books. For older children, you could play a card or board game, look at some books or just talk about topics such as favourite games, hobbies or interesting events. You can analyse the taped language sample using the procedures described in Appendix A. Each two-word utterance produced by the child can be classified in terms of the 10 rules listed earlier.

From the information collected by any or all the procedures described here, you will have clear information about the rules that the child is using now. This will enable you to plan which rules you should begin to teach.

Structured assessment of combinations of two or more words

Although you will probably be able to find out which two-word rules the child is expressing from the unstructured observational procedures just described, you may also try to elicit some two-word or longer combinations through structured activities, such as a game with pictures.

Will the child label a picture using two words? Collect a variety of pairs of pictures that have objects, people or animals that the child will recognize and can name. Try to find pairs of pictures that differ on at least one attribute, for example:

- a red car and a blue car
- a big ball and a little ball
- a glass full of milk and an empty glass
- a boy eating and a boy asleep
- a man in a car and a man in a boat
- a little dog and a big dog
- a woman sitting and a woman standing.

If possible, collect pictures that represent each of the 10 rules. Spread the pictures, in pairs, between you and the child. Say: 'Let's play a game. We can each have a turn and take a picture. I'm going to start. I want the blue car.' Take the picture with the blue car and begin your pile. Now say to the child 'Your turn. You say which one you want'. Prompt if necessary. Encourage the child to select a picture. If the child does not label it using two words or more, provide a model. Prompt the child by saying: 'you say, boy eat' or 'boy sleep' while pointing to the relevant card. Accept any utterances, but encourage the child to use at least two words. Put your fingers on the picture until the child attempts to say something. If no attempt is made after three prompts, you say the words and let the child take the picture. Now have your turn. Continue until all the pictures are gone. Record all relevant child utterances. You may find it appropriate to use a tape recorder for this. The object of this game is to elicit a variety of combinations of two or more words from the child. As in the unstructured observation tasks described previously, you can classify all the child's utterances in terms of the 10 rules listed earlier.

Once you have collected information about the word combinations that the child has produced, check these results to find out which rules have been learned and which do not yet appear to have been mastered. Some information on the rules that Jane used during both unstructured observations and the structured picture game is summarized in Table 9.3.

Table 9.3 Jane's two-word list: number of instances and percentage use of two-word rules

Rules	Number of instances	Percentage of use
Agent + action	15	31
Action + object	12	25
Agent + object	6	13
Modifier (possession) + object	2	4
Modifier (recurrence) + object	1	2
Modifier (attribution) + object	0	–
Agent/object + location	4	8
Action + location	8	17
Negation + any word	0	–
Introducer + any word	0	–

Jane is using mainly the agent + action and action + object rules. More practice could be given in using the emerging agent + object and action + location combinations such as 'dolly shoe' and 'go there'. A few examples of agent + object, modifier (possession and recurrence) + object and agent/object/action + location were observed, but no instances of the other three rules occurred in Jane's assessments. She could probably be encouraged, first, to use the action + object and agent + object rules more often, but to do this she will need a greater variety of agent, action and object words. The following sections of this chapter describe procedures that can be used to help a child like Jane to extend the combinations of two or more words that she is using.

Suggestions for encouraging early sentences

Find out if the child is expanding the meaning of the single words that are being used by adding a gesture or other action. For example, the child who pulls a toy car away from another child shouting 'car' and pointing to himself is probably trying to indicate possession. The child could be prompted to use 'my car'. This is the modifier (possession) + object rule. The child who wants you to throw, roll or kick the ball, and merely gestures while saying 'ball' could be encouraged to say 'kick ball'. This is the action + object rule. However, try to introduce only one rule at a time, as each one is a new skill for the child to master. If you are not sure which rule to introduce first, follow the order of the rules listed earlier. Most children use the agent + action and action + object rules first.

Games and activities for encouraging early sentences

A child can be helped to combine words during normal daily activities, or in games with objects or pictures. For example, during regular daily routines and periods of play with a ball or soft toys, encourage the child who is already using agent, action or object words to begin to label what is happening with two-word sentences. Instead of saying just one word, prompt the child to say two, as in 'car stop', 'push car', 'teddy eat', 'wash teddy', 'ball gone'. Model appropriate two-word phrases during routine activities; 'pants on', 'brush hair', 'wash hands', 'eat bickie'. Prompt by asking the child what is happening or what he would like to do. Some example are given in Table 9.4.

Table 9.4 Prompting for word combinations

Adult	Child	Rule
'What is happening?'	'Car gone'	Agent + action
	'Mummy car'	Agent + object
	'Puppy drink'	Agent + action
'What are you doing?'	'Ride bike'	Action + object
	'Me jump'	Agent + action
'What do you want to do?'	'Cut paper'	Action + object
	'Feed dolly'	Action + object
	'Brush hair'	Action + object
'What shall we do now?'	'Mummy bickie'	Agent + object

Developing 'scripts' for recurring events

Good opportunities for encouraging early sentences occur during routine events and activities. For example, daily routines can be used to prompt early sentences:

- Dressing: ask the child what clothes he wants to wear today, or what to put on next ('blue shirt', 'new pants')
- Meal or snack-times: encourage the child to tell you what to do next, or what she will eat next ('cut bread', 'pour juice', 'eat apple')
- Bath time: let the child choose what to wash next ('wash tummy', 'wash toes')
- Story time: ask the child 'what shall we do now?', 'turn page?', 'read book?', 'bed time?', 'light off?'

By using similar questions each time you do the same activity, and prompting a response using the binary-choice strategy, such as 'do you want blue shirt or red shirt?', or the C-I-C procedure when necessary (see

Chapter 8), the child will soon learn a variety of appropriate responses. These can then be used as a basis for new sentences with different agents, actions and objects. The predicability of these situations helps the child to remember appropriate utterances and be less dependent on your prompting and modelling of suitable phrases.

As discussed in Chapter 3, conversational routines or utterances that recur in a predictable way during daily or frequently occurring events, such as those described above, are sometimes referred to as 'scripts'. Greetings such as 'How do you do?' or 'How are you?' and the reply 'I'm fine, thanks' or 'I'm very well, thank you. How are you?' are good examples of conversational scripts that children must eventually learn. Other examples of scripts for events that most children experience often can be easily identified. For example, birthday parties have some elements that all children learn to expect; the greeting on arrival, 'Happy birthday '(child's name)' accompanied by the giving of a present; the birthday cake accompanied by singing 'Happy Birthday To You'; and the farewell of 'Bye bye' or 'Good bye. Thank you for inviting me' or 'Thank you for the present'.

One of the ways we can help children acquire language skills is by encouraging them to practise the language scripts used in recurring events such as a birthday party, a visit to the dentist (greeting, sit in the chair, open your mouth), going shopping (arrive, select items to buy, pay the money, go out) and so on. Children who attend an early childhood programme (preschool, nursery school or crèche) can learn the language associated with these familiar events during imaginative play in the 'home corner' or while dressing up. Other opportunities arise during snack-time and lunch, while using the bathroom, during story and music times, in 'home corner', blocks and outdoor play. In all these activities, children learn an appropriate script, including both actions and words. You can help children adjust to new settings by familiarizing them with the relevant scripts. These skills can also be taught at home, before the child participates in such programmes.

Structured games for using early sentences

You can help a child begin to combine words by setting up games that include opportunities for the child to label instances of the early rules. For example, the child could play with the gone box described in Chapter 7. Collect a set of objects that you know the child can label, and a box that is big enough to hold them. Cut a hole in the top of the box big enough to fit the objects into, and let the child post each object in the hole, labelling it and adding 'gone' as it disappears. Phrases such as 'cup gone', 'spoon gone', 'teddy gone' can be learned as each object is posted. As an alternative, the child can learn to say 'bye cup', 'bye spoon', 'bye teddy' as the objects are put into the gone box. Use of an appropriate gesture in conjunction with the word 'gone' or 'bye' may also act as a signal to the child that a word should be said. At first, you will need to prompt and model the correct words. Once the child has learned the rules of the game, you should not let the objects be posted until two words have been produced.

To encourage the agent + action rule, collect a series of pictures that show one agent, such as a boy or a girl, in a variety of action situations such as eating, running, washing and so on. Your aim is to encourage the child to describe what is happening in the pictures with phrases such as 'boy eat', 'boy run', 'boy wash', 'girl paint', 'girl brush', 'girl sleep'. Alternatively, select one action with different agents, as in 'Daddy sleep', 'Mummy sleep', 'puppy sleep', 'duck sleep'. Look at the pictures with the child and, if necessary, ask 'what's happening?'. Use the C-I-C strategy to elicit a two-word response. Introduce a different agent, such as 'Mummy' or 'man', using a different set of pictures, or different action words. You can find appropriate sets of pictures in early reading books, or make your own book using pictures cut out of magazines. Try to select general agent words that the child can use in many situations, but you can also encourage the use of names of familiar people, such as Nanna, Grandpa, Sam and so on. Once the child appears to have learned to use these two-word phrases without a model, listen carefully to see whether the words are also used during other daily activities. If you hear the child use examples of the types of two-word phrases you have been teaching without having just heard a model, you can assume that the rule has been mastered. Now you can select another rule and begin to teach its use.

Taking the next step

When the child is using most of the two-word sentence rules, you can begin to encourage extension into three- or four-word sentences. For instance, the child using 'push car' and 'boy push' could be encouraged to produce 'boy push car', or the child saying 'Mummy go' could be encouraged to say 'Mummy go car' or 'Mummy go home'. The important point to remember is that children can be encouraged to extend their early sentences to include another element, following the sequence listed for the two-word utterances (Table 9.5).

Table 9.5 Extension to three-word phrases

Rule	Example
Agent + action + object	'Girl push car'
Agent + action + location	'Boy go there'
Action + modifier + object	'Push big car'
Negation + action + object	'No push car'
Introducer + agent + object	'Bye Mummy car'

Programme level 5

Extending meaning: using English grammatical morphemes

At about the same time as children are learning to use all the rules for combining words into sentences, they are also beginning to take the next step in extending meaning by using grammatical morphemes to denote tense, mood and number. For example, action words are extended to indicate present and past tense, as in 'walk-ing' (present progressive), 'walk-ed' (regular past) and 'walk-s' (regular third person present). Similarly, location is identified by using prepositions such as 'in' and 'on', and plurality and possession by adding a final 's' to labelling words, as in 'dogs' and 'dog's'.

What is a morpheme? A morpheme is a word or part of a word that carries meaning. Many words can be broken down into smaller units that can be used to convey meaning. For example, 'walked' has two morphemes and can be split into 'walk-' and '-ed'. The meaning of the two parts can be recognized if the units are strung together (Owens, 1996). On the other hand, 'hot' can only be broken into 'h-' and '-ot' or 'ho-' and '-t', and these units are meaningless. Grammatical morphemes such as the present progressive '-ing', the regular past '-ed' and the plural '-s' or '-es' are described as 'bound' in that they function as markers or tags that are used to change the meaning when attached to a word. Other grammatical morphemes such as 'in', 'on', 'a' and 'the' are described as 'free' because they can stand alone, modifying another word but not attached to it. The distinction between bound and free morphemes becomes important when the length of a child's utterances is being counted. A decision may need to be made about whether to count the number of words used by the child, or the number of morphemes. For example, 'The bird is singing' has four words, but five morphemes. This issue is relevant for language assessment. Counting morphemes gives a more fine-grained analysis of progress than counting words.

Like other children, the child with delayed language usually learns to extend the meaning expressed in early sentences by adding morphemes to words, but often does this at a much slower rate than other children. Therefore, when working with such a child, it may be useful to know the sequential order in which children usually acquire grammatical morphemes in English. A list of Brown's 14 grammatical morphemes (Brown, 1973) and their order of acquisition is set out in Table 9.6. In the remaining section of this chapter, suggestions are made for assessing the child's use of grammatical morphemes by both unstructured observation and structured assessment activities. Ideas are also included for experiences that should expand the number of morphemes used by children.

Table 9.6 Brown's 14 grammatical morphemes and their order of acquisitions

Morphemes	Specific form(s)	Order of acquisition
Present progressive	-ing	1
Prepositions	In, on	2-3
Plural (regular)	-s, -es, etc.	4
Past-irregular	Came, ran, etc.	5
Possessive	-'s	6
Uncontractible copula	is, am, are, (as in: 'she is pretty')	7
Articles	a, the	8
Past regular	-d, -ed, -/t/	9
Third person regular	-s, -/z/, etc. (as in 'She runs')	10
Third person irregular	Does, has (as in: 'They do' vs. 'She does')	11
Uncontractible auxiliary	Is, am, are (as in: 'They are running')	12
Contractible copula	-'s, -'m, -'re (e.g. 'She's pretty')	13
Contractible auxiliary	-'s, -'m, -'re (e.g. 'They're running')	14

From McLean and Snyder-McLean (1978).

Unstructured assessment of grammatical morphemes

In order to find out which morphemes the child is using, you need a record of the child's actual words. If a specific morpheme is used in at least four out of five possible instances, then the child may be considered to have mastered its usage. Morphemes that occur less frequently are regarded as emerging and can be encouraged next. Opportunities can be provided later to encourage use of morphemes which are not evident or cannot be elicited. If a targeted morpheme does not emerge after practice, check to see if the child comprehends the underlying concepts. You may find that your practice sessions are more successful if you precede each session with a game in which the meaning of the target morpheme is demonstrated.

You do not need to attempt to teach all 14 of the morphemes that are included in Table 9.6, nor should the order in which they are presented in the table be strictly followed. Rather, begin by selecting one that will best help the child to communicate more effectively. Alternatively, select a morpheme that is already emerging. This would include any morpheme that is used only occasionally. You can record the morphemes that the child is using, or those that appear to be emerging, in the summary assessment sheet for morphemes that is included in Appendix B.

Information on the grammatical morphemes currently used by the child may be obtained from language samples and reports from parents, other carers or teachers. This may involve taping or video-recording the child's speech during a play session (see Appendix A), or asking parents or other carers to record the child's utterances over a set time period such as one day a week. You may wish to use the sample observational record form for recording two- or three-word utterances for this purpose or the summary assessment sheet for English morphemes in Appendix B (Level 5).

Structured assessment of grammatical morphemes

As opportunities to use all the morphemes do not always occur naturally, it is helpful to try to elicit them during a planned activity. You may find that the child is able to use certain morphemes, even though they were not evident in your observational records. In the following discussion, suggestions are made for activities that will provide the child with an opportunity to use some of the 14 grammatical morphemes identified by Brown (1973). Since not all the morphemes readily lend themselves to such elicitation, only those that can be expected to appear early in the child's development will be covered here. These include the present progressive -ing, as in 'running'; prepositions such as 'in' and 'on'; the possessive -'s as in 'Mary's shoes' and the past irregular such as 'fell', and 'sat'.

Present progressive ('-ing')

Will the child use '-ing' (the present progressive tense) with verbs to convey continuous action? Select 10 actions. Mime each action, then ask the child 'what am I doing?' If necessary prompt with 'I'm ea(t) . . . '. Suggested actions could include: eating, drinking, clapping, brushing, driving, sleeping, reading, walking, hitting, drawing, painting. Does the child use '-ing' appropriately?

If the child uses '-ing' in four out of five of the responses, then this morpheme has been acquired. If '-ing' is not used at the required level, you will need to give more practice in this skill. If '-ing' is not used at all, model the answer and encourage the child to imitate you. Then demonstrate at least three of the actions again and ask 'What am I doing?' Does the child use '-ing' after modelling?

If yes, you can conclude that more practice is likely to be helpful. If no, then the child may not yet be ready to extend his or her language in this way.

Suggestions for encouraging use of the present progressive ('-ing')
Collect some simple pictures of actions, such as a boy jumping, a woman kissing a baby, a dog running and a girl eating an ice-cream. If the child's normal response when asked 'tell me what is happening' is to say 'boy jump', then model and prompt the response 'boy jumping', using the C-I-C strategy. If the child says 'kiss baby', you should encourage use of 'kissing baby' and so on. You could also use action games, with the adult miming actions and then asking. 'What am I doing?' Alternatively, use dolls or soft toys to demonstrate the actions in a game. Take turns with the child to model an action and then ask 'What's doll doing?' or 'Tell me what teddy is doing'. The binary choice strategy of asking, for example, 'is

the boy swimming or jumping?' may also be useful in the beginning because it provides the child with cues about how to answer.

The morpheme 'in'

Will the child use 'in' to define the location of an object? Give the child five opportunities to answer a question such as 'where is the ball?', using 'in' + 'there', or 'in' + a labelling word. You will need to collect five small containers such as a cup, box, shoe, bag and a toy car or truck and a small ball. Let the child watch you hide the ball in one of the five containers. Ask 'Where's the ball?'. Try not to let the child substitute pointing or another gestural response, by making sure both hands are away, either folded away or held by you. Alternatively, close your eyes and say 'Tell me where'. Repeat the task with each of the containers. Does the child use 'in' appropriately?

If 'in' is used in four out of five of the responses, then you can assume that this morpheme has been acquired. If it is not used at the required level, you will need to devise some games to encourage this skill.

If the child did not use 'in', model the answer 'in the bag' or 'in the shoe' and encourage imitation as you repeat the five tasks. Does the child use 'in' after modelling?

If yes, you can conclude that this skill is emerging and some practice in use of the morpheme can be given. If no, the child is probably not yet ready to learn to use this morpheme.

Suggestions for encouraging use of 'in'

Collect an assortment of pictures showing items inside a variety of containers. Show them to the child and label each picture; for example, 'juice in a cup', 'Daddy in his bed', 'bottle in her mouth', 'baby in the pram', 'bird in a nest'. By using the C-I-C strategy, the child has the opportunity to learn the response needed to answer a question such as 'Where's the baby?' with the answer 'in pram' or 'in the pram'.

During normal daily activities, ask the child where common household objects belong; for example, in the bath or cupboard or bin. Once again, use the C-I-C or a binary choice strategy.

The morpheme 'on'

Will the child use 'on' to define the location of an object?

Prepare five pairs of objects that can be arranged so that one is supported on top of the other. Examples might include a doll or yourself with a hat on; a spoon balancing on a cup; a toy car on a box; a doll on a chair and a ball on a book. Ask 'Where's . . . ?'. If necessary, encourage the child by asking 'tell me where'. Each answer should be 'on + . . . ' or 'on there'. Does the child use 'on' appropriately?

If the child uses 'on' in four out of five responses, you can assume that this morpheme has been acquired. If not, you will need to plan more games to practise this skill. To find out whether the child will use 'on' after modelling, repeat the five tasks, but model the answer in each case, and encourage the child to imitate you. Does the child use 'on' after it has been modelled?

If yes, you can conclude that the child will benefit from more practice in the use of 'on'. If no, it is probably not yet appropriate to help the child in this way.

Suggestion for practising use of 'on'
Tell the child that you are going to put an object, such as a car, 'on' various things and you want her to say where it is. You could even put the child 'on' the table', a chair', a big ball' or use a doll or other object to demonstrate 'on'. Remember to use the C-I-C or binary choice strategies in these activities.

Once the child has learned the rules of the game, you should change roles. Let the child try to trick you by putting an object 'on' something unexpected. Look for opportunities during the day to practise use of this word.

The plural -s

Will the child indicate number (plurality) by adding a final -s to object labels? Collect a shoe-box or drawstring bag and put several similar or identical objects in it. Hand the child the box or bag and say 'Look. What's in here?' The answer should be ' . . . -s' as in 'cows', 'keys' and 'spoons'. Repeat this for five different objects. Some appropriate items to use include spoons, cups, cars, balls and blocks. Does the child add the final '-s' to the object labels?

If the plural -s is used in four out of five instances, then the child has acquired its use. However, if the plural -s is not used at the required level, the child will need more practice. If there is no evidence of usage of the plural -s, you should repeat the task, but model the appropriate answer and encourage imitation. Does the child use the plural '-s' after modelling?

If yes, then you can conclude that he will probably benefit from more practice.

Remember to provide some opportunities for the child to understand the concept of plurality before you introduce a model of the morpheme for imitation. This will help him learn to use it appropriately.

Suggestions for encouraging use of the regular plural -s
Assemble collections of items such as pencils, blocks, buttons and a box. Take turns with the child to tell each other to 'put the buttons in the box' and so on. Or you could collect pairs of pictures, one of each pair showing a single object, the other showing several examples of the same object. Give the child one of the pair and keep the other. Label the picture 'car', 'cars'; 'apple', 'apples'; 'cat', 'cats' as appropriate. Once again, use the C-I-C or binary choice strategies.

It is a good idea to avoid irregular plural forms (such as sheep and feet) when the child is learning this morpheme. These can be acquired later.

Past irregular tense

Will the child demonstrate use of the past tense of irregular action words such as broke, fell, ran, sat, blew? Demonstrate a series of actions such as those listed below, using dolls, cars, animals or any toy that moves or changes. Afterwards ask 'what happened?' or 'what did I do?' or 'what did dolly do?'. The child should reply using the past irregular tense if she is able to mark with words the time aspect of the event.

The following are some possible action sequences:

fell   a doll walks and then falls down
ran   a doll runs
sat   show doll sitting on a chair, then remove the chair
blew   blow out a match or candle or blow a light object such as a
       feather
broke   show a sharp pencil point, then break it or break a twig in half.

Does the child comment on the events using the past tense of an irregular verb? If the child used the past irregular in four out of five responses, you can assume that he is able to represent past tense in this manner. If not, more opportunities to practise may be needed. Repeat the demonstrations but model the correct answers and encourage the child to imitate them. Does the child use the past irregular after modelling?

If yes, then the child will probably profit from more encouragement in using this form. If no, then the child is probably not yet ready to learn to express the past irregular verb form.

Suggestions for encouraging use of the past irregular form of action words
Play a series of games with objects that provide opportunities for use of past irregular verb forms. Model the word and encourage the child to imitate. Use a series of picture cards that demonstrate these action sequences, such as Jack and Jill or Humpty Dumpty. Ask 'what happened?', then 'what happened next?'.

The possessive (-'s)

Will the child indicate possession by using the '-'s' with labelling words? Select items that are known to belong to five members of the family or playmates, such as bags, shoes, hats or toys. Ask 'whose is this?', or 'who does this belong to?' Does the child indicate possession with '-'s'?

If the child used the possessive '-'s' in four out of five instances, she has this skill. If it is used inconsistently, more practice is needed. If there is no evidence of use of '-'s', repeat the tasks, but model the answer each time and encourage the child to imitate. For example, point to the child's pants/shoe/chair and ask 'whose is this?' and answer '(Tom)'s pants/shoe/chair'. Does the child use a possessive '-'s' after modelling?

If yes, you should give more practice. If no, the child is probably not yet ready to learn to use this speech form.

Suggestions for encouraging the possessive ('-'s')

Have paper dolls or pictures of a boy and girl and let the child sort out pictures of clothes that belong to each. As the clothes are sorted, use the C-I-C or binary choice strategy to elicit the correct response. You should label each item as 'boy's . . . ' or 'girl's . . . ', allowing the child a turn to sort or dress the doll when the possessive marker is used appropriately.

Alternatively, select a colourful picture of a dog (or another animal) and as you point to the body parts, label 'dog's tail', 'dog's nose' and so on. Encourage the child to imitate. Once again, the C-I-C and binary choice strategies can be used.

Other morphemes

The remaining morphemes (the last eight in Brown's list) have not been discussed in detail here because they are usually acquired later, when the child has more advanced language skills. However, they may also be encouraged through games that involve objects and pictures, or at appropriate times during normal daily activities.

Children who are slow in acquiring the early morphemes sometimes do not attend to speech closely enough to perceive small sounds such as '-s', '-ing' or '-ed' when they are embedded in a longer utterance. It may be helpful to include some activities that will help the child learn to listen more carefully to the speech that is heard as part of a language programme. Games such as 'Simon Says' can help a child learn to listen. Similarly, any activity that includes an action that is contingent on hearing a morpheme can be used. For example, give the child a page with drawings of balloons. Let the child colour in a balloon when a morpheme that you are currently practising is heard. For example:

dog running   colour a balloon
dog run   do not colour a balloon

Other possible games include bingo, where the child puts a coloured counter on a card each time the morpheme is heard. A postbox game can also be used in which the child 'posts' a counter each time the target morpheme is heard. Activities like these will help the child attend to the morphemes that are embedded in speech.

It is important to remember that morphemes are often acquired very slowly, because children probably need to develop an understanding of the underlying concepts before they can be expected to use morphemes correctly. When providing activities to encourage the use of particular morphemes, it is a good idea to begin the session with some games that demonstrate the meaning of the morpheme that you want to teach. In normal language development in English-speaking children, in terms of the child's mean length of utterance, the pattern of acquisition occurs in the following sequence shown in Table 9.7.

Table 9.7 Mean length of utterance: pattern of acquisition

Mean length of utterance	Morphemes acquired
2.0–2.5	-ing; in; on
2.5–3.0	Past irregular; possessive (-'s); uncontracted copula
3.0–3.7	Articles; regular past; third-person regular; third-person irregular uncontracted
3.7–4.5	Auxiliary; contracted copula; contracted progressive auxiliary

Once children have learned to use grammatical morphemes they are able to convey more complex meanings such as number and tense. They will continue to refine these messages, with the addition of other forms and constructions from the adult grammatical system, until they have acquired the range of skills that are present in the speech of mature language users.

Summary

There is some evidence that children who have been delayed in producing first words will show further delay in combining words into simple phrases and sentences. This chapter suggests ways for assessing the language skills of children who are using single words and for encouraging them to combine words according to the 10 two-word rules. This development represents an important step towards learning to express meaning in more complex phrases and sentences.

By the time that children have acquired the principal grammatical morphemes of their language community, it may be said that the skills that contribute to becoming a competent language user have been mastered. Once this level is reached, your task should be to ensure that opportunities to use language skills appropriately are provided with peers as well as adult partners. In this way, the child will learn that talking is worthwhile, both as a social tool and as a means for making things happen.

Once children begin to produce three- and four-word utterances, you will need to consider one additional aspect of their language: pragmatics or the communicative intentions that are expressed through actions, gestures, sounds and words. This aspect of language should be monitored throughout the language acquisition process since communicative intentions will be evident from the time that children first begin to use their actions and vocalizations to communicate with their carers. This aspect of communication is considered in the next chapter.

Chapter 10
Communicative intentions

Many people associate the beginning of real communication with children's use of consistent sounds and words to represent specific events or activities. However, intentional communication starts even earlier. It can be observed when infants reach out and grasp, tug, point or use other gestures and actions to communicate their interests or needs to significant other people in their environment. These early behaviours represent the pragmatic function of language and communication (Bates, O'Connell and Shore, 1987; Reichle, Halle and Johnson, 1993; Wetherby, Warren and Reickle, 1998). Early forms of communicative intent can be observed in the actions, and sounds of very young infants who are acquiring the preliminary skills that underlie language. These early pragmatic behaviours are used to draw a carer's attention to something of interest, request a desired object, control another's actions or interact socially. Evidence of their emergence can be observed in the preverbal communicative behaviour of children at levels 1–3 in the language programme (see Table 10.1). As more advanced verbal skills are acquired, children who are at programme levels 4 and 5 and can use sentences begin to express more complex pragmatic functions such as asking and answering questions, finding new words and giving information.

Table 10.1 Levels in children's intentional communication

Level	Communicative intentions
1–3	Indicate or comment
	Obtain or request
	Regulate: protest, reject, request attention, and social interaction
4–5	Use words to express intentions; ask questions
	Discover new words; give information; answer questions

Communicative intentions can be observed when children attract attention, indicate the presence of a familiar object or person, or achieve a desired outcome through a variety of actions, gestures and sounds. The sounds used in these early communicative acts sometimes take the form of performatives or protowords (see Chapter 2). For example, as morning snack-time approaches Kate (aged around 18 months) goes to the kitchen and reaches towards the cupboard where the biscuits are kept, while looking towards her mother who interprets these actions as communicating that the baby wants something to eat. As her father enters the room, Kate looks up, beams and bounces up and down where she is sitting. Dad interprets her actions as indicating recognition and attention. He goes to pick her up. In this way the child's family observes and interprets her actions or gestures, attaching meaning to them and responding appropriately. This encourages Kate to continue communicating her wants even though she is not yet able to use consistent sounds or words.

The ability to communicate our wants to others is an important *pragmatic* or social skill. Most children learn very rapidly that specific gestures, with or without accompanying sounds, evoke particular responses from familiar adults and they begin to use them often during daily activities to signal their interests and needs. Such signals are usually maintained until the child's goal is achieved. These early communicative intentions typically involve other people and are idiosyncratic in their expression, varying from child to child. Careful observation of children's non-verbal intentional communicative behaviour enables familiar adults to recognize the intended meaning and respond appropriately. Children who are slow to develop vocal skills usually acquire an array of consistent actions for communicating their intentions. Such children can be helped to increase their intentional communication skills through systematic encouragement and refinement of their actions and gestures (Warren and Yoder, 1998).

Children who are slow to communicate intentionally using gestures, sounds or words can sometimes be assisted to express these meanings by using non-verbal means. For example, children who have appropriate receptive language and fine motor skills but are not yet using words to indicate their interests may respond to the use of signs to assist in their communication. Use of a system of signs and other forms of augmentative communication is discussed in Chapter 12.

Early communicative intentions: the social use of language

The early actions, gestures and sounds produced by children generally have a social function and are used to signal a communicative intent to a familiar adult. Many researchers have attempted to identify the functions present in children's early communicative behaviour, based on interpretation of infant actions by an observer. There is some variation in the taxonomies or sets of functions that have been described. For example, Reichle, Halle and Johnson (1993, pp. 110–114) list the different taxonomies of communicative intent described by Dore (1975), Coggins and Carpenter (1978), Cirrin and Rowland (1985) and Wetherby and Prizant (1989). Halliday (1973, 1975) was one of the first to propose a set of categories to describe the function of early communication based on observation of his son. According to Halliday's analysis, infants and toddlers use their actions and sounds to:

- *Indicate* or *comment* on the existence of a person, object or event: for example, by looking or reaching towards a familiar adult or area of interest (cupboard, toy), holding out a toy towards a familiar person or looking towards an adult when a familiar song or tune is heard or a familiar character appears on the television.
- *Obtain* or *request* a desired object or service: for example, reaching towards or banging on cupboard to get a favourite toy or lifting arms to be picked up.
- *Regulate* other people's actions:
  - *protest*, as in an angry cry when an interesting object is removed
  - *rejection*, as in pushing away unwanted food or toy, putting head down to avoid taking part in activity or turning away from an adult or activity
  - *requesting attention*, as in tugging at adult's leg, reaching towards adult, bouncing up and down on spot as adult enters field of vision
- *Initiate, maintain or terminate social interaction*, as in bringing a toy or book to an adult, continuing to rock back and forth even though the adult has stopped rocking, or turning or moving away from a joint play activity.

It is important to remember that although there are similarities between the actions or gestures used by children to signal their communicative intentions, there are variations in the means used by different children. Each child needs to be carefully observed to determine the specific intentions embedded in a particular behaviour.

Most infants learn to recognize the sounds, words and actions produced by adults when they respond to primitive communicative acts. Over time, as efforts to communicate increase, they will attempt to reproduce these sounds, words and actions intentionally. However, families of children whose communication development is delayed can be slow to 'read' the connection between a child's gestures or actions and the intended message. Their lack of feedback exacerbates the children's problems. Such children can be helped to learn to use their gestures and sounds to satisfy their needs, both by sensitizing parents to the meaning of a child's behaviour and by enhancing the 'readability' of the child's communicative actions. The focus of the following discussion is on helping children to make the meaning of their communicative attempts clearer.

Suggested assessment activities

Children's communicative intentions can be assessed by careful observation over a period of time and in a variety of both structured and unstructured situations. The aim of such observation is to find out which of the early communicative intentions (indicating, requesting, regulating and initiating) is being expressed by the child. If you are not able to observe the child informally, suggestions about situations that can be used for structured assessment are described below. A checklist with these early intentions is included in the summary assessment sheets in Appendix B. Use this summary sheet to record the results of your assessment. Use the level 2 sheet for communicative intentions if the child is using actions, gestures or sounds to communicate, and the level 5 sheet if the child is using single words, signs, phrases or sentences.

Here are some suggestions for assessing whether the child is regularly communicating intentions using actions or gestures.

Unstructured observation of early communicative intentions

Observe the child in a variety of natural settings. Watch to see whether the child is using any actions or gestures to attract your attention to communicate his or her wants. Make a list of any actions and gestures that you see. Note when they occur and the meaning that you think is intended. Note also the mode that is used; action, gesture, sound or word. You can also ask parents, carers or other familiar adults which meanings the child is expressing and the manner in which they are expressed (by actions, gestures, sounds or words). In addition, provided you have the facilities and are able to obtain the family's approval, you may find the most effective way to assess communicative intentions is to video the child in a variety of informal group settings during the day at home, at preschool or at playgroup.

Structured assessment of early communicative intentions

Since the production of communicative intentions is totally under the control of the child, it can be difficult to devise situations in which these behaviours can be elicited for the purpose of assessment. If you decide to use the structured assessment tasks described here, be aware that children may fail to respond appropriately because they do not want to comply rather than because they have not yet learned to use language in these ways.

Here are some suggestions for assessing the first three pragmatic functions identified earlier (indicating, obtaining and regulating). Assessing the fourth function (initiation, maintenance and termination of social interaction) is best done through observation.

Indicating the existence of people, objects or events

Does the child show you things that are of particular interest? Does she:

- reach and grasp, point, gesture or make a sound to attract your attention or the attention of others to look at something of interest?

- attempt to point out something of interest to an adult?
- indicate the existence of an interesting object?

Take a number of familiar objects and sit down with the child in a comfortable position on the floor or at a table. As you prepare to play, 'accidentally' push an object away from you and the child. Ignore the incident. Does the child draw your attention to it? If yes, how does he communicate – by action, gesture, sound or word? At the end of the activity, pack the objects into a box, leaving one out. Does the child draw your attention to the forgotten object? How?

Does the child indicate the existence of a person? Observe the child's reaction as you approach. Does the child look towards you and indicate recognition in any way? If possible, have another person enter the room. Does the child look towards the other person then back to you? Does the child gesture in any way to indicate recognition of the other person?

Does the child indicate the existence of an interesting event? Sit with the child and quietly start playing a familiar tune on a tape (you could also use a musical toy). Ignore the music. Note whether the child tries to draw your attention to it. How?

If the child draws your attention in one or more of these situations, you may conclude that he knows how to indicate something to another person.

Obtaining objects or services

Will the child attempt to obtain the assistance of another person to get something that she wants? Does she use an appropriate skill to do this? Collect four small toys that interest the child. Place them slightly out of her reach. Push the first toy towards the child until she takes it. Now let her know that she can have the remaining toys. When the child has difficulty reaching the second toy, offer to help. When you have helped the child to obtain this toy, indicate that she should also take the other toys. This time do not help unless she uses an action, gesture, sound or word to obtain assistance. Does the child try to obtain your help? How?

Show the child three favourite toys that can be seen but are out of reach. Take one toy and give it to the child or lift the child to reach the toy. Now indicate that the child can have the second toy. If the child does not use a gesture, action, sound or word to obtain assistance to reach the toy, indicate that you are willing to assist. When the child has this toy, indicate that he can have the other. This time, do not offer assistance unless he uses an action, gesture, word or sound to obtain help. If the child responds in either situation, you may conclude that he knows how to obtain help from another person.

Regulating other people's actions – protest, reject, request attention

This intention is difficult to assess formally. However, if you are unable to observe it informally, the following is a suggestion that you may be able to use:

- *Protest*: While the child is playing with an object, attempt to take it away. Does the child use an appropriate action, gesture, sound or word to protest?
- *Rejection*: Offer the child an object that you know she does not usually like. Does the child use an appropriate action, gesture, sound or word to indicate rejection of the object?
- *Request attention*: ask an adult who is familiar to the child to come and sit close to her. The adult should avoid looking at the child. Does the child use a gesture, action, sound or word to indicate that she wants the adult's attention?

If the child responds appropriately to two of these situations, you may conclude that she knows how to regulate other people's actions.

Initiating, maintaining and terminating social interaction

The pragmatic functions associated with social interaction are best assessed informally. However, you may be able to use the following suggestions in a formal situation.

As the child enters a room, sit playing with a toy or engaged in an activity that you expect the child to enjoy and which can be used in a turn-taking game. Examples include drawing, blowing bubbles.

- Does the child come up to you and use an appropriate action, gesture, sound or word to attract your attention?
- If you stop playing, does the child indicate with a gesture, action, sounds or words that she wishes you to continue?
- Does she use a gesture, action, sound or word at any time to indicate that the game is no longer of interest?
- Does the child use any action, gesture sound or word to attract your attention when you come into a room?
- Does the child wave on leaving the room or if you say 'bye bye' or indicate in some other way that you are leaving.

If the child indicates his intention appropriately in at least two of these situations, you may conclude that he knows how to regulate social interaction.

Once you have collected information through observation or structured assessment about the child's use of gestures, actions, sounds or words to express intentions, you can decide whether it is necessary to provide experiences that will encourage more effective expression of these meanings. For example, if the child uses several different sounds along with gestures to tell you something, attract your attention or reject it, you may wish to combine helping her to communicate specific intentions with the use of performative sounds (see Chapter 7). If, however, the child is able to attract your attention or indicate her wants only by screaming, stamping or other inappropriate actions, you will need to introduce more acceptable means to express these intentions. For example, the child could learn to put arms up to indicate 'please pick me up', pat the lid of the biscuit container to request a biscuit or put out an open hand to request a toy. In the following sections, suggestions are made for games and other activities that can be used to assist children to communicate these intentions more effectively. As with all early communication skills, these are best introduced as part of a game or when appropriate opportunities occur during the day.

Suggestions for encouraging communicative intentions

The primary objective here is to help children acquire skills that can be used to influence and control aspects of their environment; for example, to gain attention and satisfy current needs. The immediate goal is to help them learn to use conventional, readily understood actions, gestures, sounds, words or intonation patterns intentionally to convey meaning. Initially, particularly with children who are acquiring the preliminary skills of looking together, taking turns and imitating, and appropriate play, you will need to concentrate on learning to communicate intentionally by using non-verbal means such as gestures or physical movements. You can accompany the child's actions with appropriate sounds or words. As the child becomes more competent, you can assist him to pair the gestures and movements with appropriate words or signs (the use of signs is discussed in Chapter 12). Many of the learning activities described in other chapters can be used here provided that the child takes an active role as initiator or leader in the game.

When introducing these activities, remember that children do not always interpret your actions in the way you intend. For example, an action such as pushing something away to indicate rejection can be interpreted by a child as acknowledgment of existence rather than as rejection. In this situation, the child may learn to push aside or apparently 'reject' desirable objects. Try to ensure that the child understands the meaning you intend for any action that you introduce.

Learning to indicate the existence of people, objects or events

Many children will tug your arm, point or reach out to indicate that they have seen something of interest. Such behaviour often occurs when the child is engaged in play with a favourite toy, or you are both looking at a book or a preferred television programme or video. Watch to see if the child uses a gesture, sound or word to indicate. If necessary, use the suggested structured assessment activities to help you. If you do not see this type of behaviour, or if the child looks towards the person or object of interest without engaging your attention too, model appropriate actions and words and encourage the child to imitate you. Your aim is to help him learn that it is worthwhile to get others to look at things that are interesting. You may need to physically assist the child to use an appropriate action or gesture. Watch for suitable situations and when the child appears to show interest in a person, picture or object, help him to indicate using the action or gesture that you have chosen. Examples can include reaching out to indicate to you that he sees a lost ball or pointing to show you the picture that he is drawing. Comment appropriately as you guide the child's movements, saying 'look', 'there', or 'it's there'.

Once the child appears to have learned the connection between a specific action or gesture and a particular communicative intention, watch to see whether it is used in suitable situations. If the child regularly uses the action or gesture to indicate the existence of people, objects or events, you can conclude that this communicative function has been acquired. If not, you may need to give more practice either by physically assisting the child or by modelling the action yourself as the child looks towards the person or object of interest and encouraging imitation.

Suitable times to assist the child to learn to indicate include occasions when:

- a familiar person walks into the room
- a favourite character or advertisement appears on the television screen
- an interesting car, truck, bus or dog passes by while you are out walking
- looking at a picture book together
- collecting flowers in the garden
- taking favourite toys out of a bag or box.

Learning to obtain desired objects or services

Obtaining desired objects or services is important to most children. If a child uses only generalized actions or noises such as kicking or screaming to obtain objects or services, it is time to introduce some more appropriate actions, gestures or sounds. Watch to find out what strategies the child is using for these purposes. If necessary, use the suggested assessment activities. If the child does not appear to use any appropriate strategies it may be useful to help him develop some specific gestures to indicate these wants. It is important to choose social situations and objects and services that are important to the child.

Once you have decided on the situations and gestures you will introduce, encourage their use when appropriate opportunities arise. For example, when the child stretches out her arms to be picked up, you say 'up?' with appropriate intonation as you pick her up. Once she appears to have learned the connection between the word and the desired object or service, watch to see whether she uses it at appropriate times. If she does, you can assume that she has learned to communicate this intention and can begin to give opportunities for learning other ways to obtain objects or services. If not, you may need to give the child more practice either by physically prompting or assisting the child or by modelling the appropriate action or gesture.

Some suitable times to assist the child to learn to obtain desired objects or services as listed in Table 10.2.

Table 10.2 Obtaining desired objects or services

To be picked up	Child raises arms together as adult says 'up'
To open a container	Child pats the lid once or twice as adult says 'open'
To have door opened	Child knocks several times as adult says 'open'
To have adult sit with child	Child taps chair or floor as adult says 'sit'
To have television on	Child touches television set as adult says 'on, TV on'
To obtain something to eat or drink	Child touches or rubs tummy as adult says 'eat/drink, you want to eat/drink'

Learning to regulate other people's actions

Learning to regulate the actions of others involves two main skills: learning to protest and reject, and learning to request attention from another person. Most children acquire these skills fairly easily, but some children experience difficulty expressing these meanings intentionally using appropriate actions or words.

Most children learn to say 'no' or 'don't' without any difficulty. However, children who are having difficulty learning to talk sometimes do not begin to use them and may not even learn to protest or reject by other means, such as crying, or turning away to avoid something they do not want. You should observe the child carefully and find out whether he or she is expressing protest or rejection by using actions, gestures, sounds or words. If necessary, use the suggested structured activities to help you. It the child does not appear to be expressing these meanings in any form you may need to devise situations in which appropriate actions and gestures can be learned.

Look for suitable opportunities to model the expression of protest and rejection through gestures and words. If necessary, set up a game in which the child can learn to communicate in this way. For example, while the child is playing with a favourite toy, take hold of it or get in the way so the child cannot continue the game. Encourage the child to push you away as you say the word 'no'. If necessary, assist the child to push you away. Then let the game continue. Repeat your action and encourage the child to copy you. Once you have observed the child expressing protest or rejection using actions spontaneously, you will know that this communicative function has been acquired.

Learning to request attention

Children usually learn to attract attention to themselves at an early age. In a busy family, this is an important skill for a child to acquire. Many children learn to say 'Mama', or its equivalent in their home language, to get attention and will later call out phrases such as 'look at me' to ensure that an adult looks when they are jumping, climbing or doing something of interest. Watch to see if the child is using actions, words or sounds to attract attention. If necessary, use the structured activities suggested earlier. If the child does not use actions to attract attention and is not yet using a variety of sounds, you could help her to clap hands to signal this intention. You can also observe carefully any sounds that the child makes and model one of these sounds vigorously as you do the action. If the child does not yet use sounds or words, it is often easier for him to learn, first, to initiate, maintain or terminate social interaction before any attempt is made to help him learn to request attention.

Learning to initiate, maintain or terminate social interaction

The skills of initiating, maintaining or terminating a social exchange are best learned in appropriate situations during the day:

- As you and the child greet another person, assist her to make an appropriate gesture such as moving one hand in a small arc across the body while saying 'hi' or 'hello'.
- When saying goodbye to another person, assist the child to wave as you say 'bye bye'. Encourage the child to use appropriate gestures to greet other family members each morning and to say goodbye to them at bedtime.
- Encourage the child to initiate and terminate interaction using the greeting and farewell actions each time she goes to school or daycare, when visiting friends and so on.
- Assist the child until you feel that she is able to do the appropriate action unaided. Continue to model the action or prompt the child as necessary until you see the gestures regularly.

To maintain social interaction, you may encourage the child to give a play partner a turn at pushing the car, or pat the knee or shoulder of the next person to indicate 'your turn' in a turn-taking activity such as looking in a surprise bag or catching bubbles. Remember to model an appropriate sound or word each time you encourage the child to use the action or gesture to communicate these socially interactive intentions.

Expressing communicative intentions using words

Once children are able to use words, they can begin to use them to regulate the behaviour of others. Ideas for assessing and encouraging development of early communicative intentions using actions and gestures are given in the first part of this chapter. These same strategies can be used to encourage the use of appropriate words to express more complex communicative functions such as asking and answering questions and discovering new words. However, to obtain information about such topics as 'what', 'when', 'where', 'why', 'how' or 'who', children usually need to have begun to use sentences of at least two words. Development of these language functions is also dependent on the child's continuing semantic development, that is, understanding the meaning of the words that are used. Once they are able to combine a number of words into simple sentences, young children usually become very interested in asking questions such as 'where Daddy?' 'Wa'sis?' and 'What this?' Some young children will continually ask 'Wha'sis?' holding up a familiar object or 'Where Mummy?' when left at grandmother's or babysitter's house. At this early stage, however, although they know what they mean, they are not aware of the syntactic rules they are using when they say 'wha'sis?' but are simply using the combined words as a single word or 'holophrase'.

Being able to take part in a conversation is essential for children if they are to join in social and group activities. It is through such interactions that much of their learning will occur. As part of the skills needed to function successfully within a group, they need to learn to use appropriate language for several purposes.

- *To obtain information by asking questions.* Initially children use intonation alone to ask questions, as in 'my drink?' Once they are able to use sentences, they start to ask by using words such as 'where . . . ?', 'what . . . ?', 'when . . . ?', 'who . . . ?', 'how . . . ?' and 'why . . . ?'.
- *To discover new words* as in 'what's this?', 'what is this?' and "what is . . . called?' This is a special form of questioning. When children use sentences of this type they are demonstrating metalinguistic awareness or an understanding of language as a system of signs and symbols. By the time children start to use this sentence form, they have usually started to use a number of early grammatical morphemes (reviewed in Chapter 9).
- *To give information* such as 'that's a . . . ' and 'it's a . . . ' as well as to request it. Children who use this function spontaneously are usually quite competent language users.
- *To answer questions* using sentences such as 'yes, I want one'. This is an important use of language because children need to be able to respond appropriately to questions directed to them. When they can use language in this way they are demonstrating some of the most important elements of a conversation, including knowledge of the rules involved in:
  - taking turns with a partner in a dyadic exchange (eye contact, proximity)
  - waiting for a turn
  - responding at the correct time

- recognizing the meaning intended by a speaker in asking a question
- understanding that an appropriate response should be produced; and
- keeping to the topic.

Children who have difficulty learning to use words and sentences often have difficulty learning to express these more complex communicative intentions verbally.

Suggested assessment activities

Observation is the best way to find out whether children are expressing their intentions by using words. Observe the child in a variety of natural settings. If necessary, ask the child's parents or other familiar adults if the child expresses any of these meanings verbally. You may like to set up some of the games or activities listed below to help you in your observations. A checklist, including a description of the eight communicative intentions you should look for, is included in the summary assessment sheets in Appendix B.

Suggestions for encouraging more complex communicative intentions

Use of appropriate syntactic forms to express these functions is best encouraged in the natural social contexts. These can occur in one-to-one situations with an adult, but they are best practised in larger group settings such as at home with the family or at preschool, nursery school and so on. Appropriate contexts can include daily routines such as meal and snack times or during structured and unstructured play. If the child is experiencing difficulty in expressing any of the syntactic forms used to express the more advanced communicative intentions, a good way to introduce them is during turn-taking games with an adult or more competent children.

Turn-taking games used to practise syntactic forms such as questioning need to be organized so that the child can take both roles, asking and answering questions. The adult should initially take the questioner role, to model it for the child. Strategies such as the C-I-C strategy and binary choice may be used to model appropriate questions and answers (these are explained in Chapter 8). The child can then be invited to change roles and question the adult. Once the rules of the game are learned, these games can be played with small groups of children, with all the children taking turns to ask as well as answer questions. Suitable games for practising these skills include:

- *lotto games*: children can take turns to ask "what's this?', 'who's got . . .?' or '(child's name), have you got . . . ?' and to answer appropriately.

Remember to begin with the simpler form of questioning and only move on to the more complicated form as the child becomes proficient in the earlier one.

- *Board and card games* that involve matching: examples include colour matching or 'match and turn' games that give opportunities for children to ask 'what . . . ?' and to respond 'it's (colour or object label)'. Once children understand the rules of the game, they can play together in small groups with more competent children providing models for those who are still developing these skills.
- *Surprise bag* (see Chapter 7): children can take turns to ask 'what have you got?', 'what's this?' or 'what's in the bag' and to answer 'I've got a . . .' or 'it's a . . .'.
- *Hiding games* can be used to encourage asking and answering of 'where . . . ?' questions and giving information about location as in 'It's in . . .' and ' . . .'s there'. Take turns with the child to hide an object and ask 'where's (object or person)'.

Remember to model a behaviour several times before expecting a child to ask the question. Alternatively, the child can play a matching card game in a small group with the child asking 'where . . . ?' rather than the more complicated 'who has . . . ?'.

Group turn-taking and circle games such as 'Doggie, Doggie Who's Got the Bone?' and 'Knock, Knock Who's There?' that repeat a single question over and over in the form of a group chant can also help children to learn to ask questions. Socio-dramatic play is another excellent context in which to practice these skills. Some scenarios that can be created include shop, restaurant, and doctor's surgery.

In all these activities, remember to encourage the child to take both questioner and respondent roles.

Summary

Learning to use language in a variety of ways to influence the actions and attention of others is a very important part of learning to talk. This is the social aspect of language and without these skills, the child is unable to communicate effectively in the social context. A child may learn to play appropriately and to use a variety of actions, gestures, sounds or words, but these skills are relatively useless if the child is not able to use them to influence events and the actions of others. These early communicative intentions are part of the pragmatic aspect of a language system. They are as important to the child who is learning to talk as are the other aspects of language (semantics, syntax, morphology and phonology). It is therefore advisable for children to learn to use their communication skills intentionally at the same time as they are learning to take turns, play appropriately and produce early sounds and words. The child who is able to signal communicative intentions adequately will usually learn to use words and sounds more readily as he or she learns that sounds and words can be used to 'make things happen'.

This concludes Part 2 of this book. The remaining chapters are concerned with some of the more general issues in language acquisition, such as increasing the intelligibility of speech, use of signs or pictorial systems to supplement speech, working with children in groups, working with children from language backgrounds other than English and working with families. These topics often need to be addressed when efforts are made to help children who are experiencing difficulties to become more competent language users.

Part 3
Issues in implementation

The final chapters of the book explore a number of practical issues associated with the provision of language development experiences for children experiencing delays and difficulties. Phonological aspects of development are addressed first by Christine Hardman, a speech pathologist with wide experience in helping children with phonological difficulties and in advising parents and other carers how to help such children. The use of signs and other forms of augmentative or alternative communication to supplement or complement prelinguistic or relatively unintelligible attempts to communicate are then examined in Chapter 12.

Issues arising from attempts to assist children experiencing language and communication problems whose language background is other than English are considered in Chapter 13. Such children are often helped to communicate more effectively while they are in group settings such as a preschool, nursery school, child care centre or playgroup, and guidelines for those working with groups of children are included in Chapter 14. Finally, in Chapter 15 suggestions are made about issues that need to be considered when working with parents who are concerned about the language development of their child and want to participate in any programme that is provided for the child.

Chapter 11
Phonological development and intelligibility

CHRISTINE A. HARDMAN, SPEECH PATHOLOGIST

Most children begin life by 'telling' us just how they are feeling, through a whimper or a lusty yell. The skill of making sounds has begun, but between the earliest cry of hunger or pain and the most complicated spoken word there is often a lengthy, sometimes bumpy, path of development and refinement. This chapter is concerned with these changes. It begins with a review of the early development of phonological skills and then provides suggestions about ways to promote children's sound making in the early stages of learning to talk.

Development of sounds

The earliest recognizable sounds of communication are varied cries representing a variety of needs or emotions. As infants become more involved with the world and begin to enjoy the noises that they can make, the sounds become more gurgling or vowel-like as in 'ah' and 'oo'. Carers will often find this behaviour very pleasurable, spending much time gurgling and cooing in response. These early sounds need little effort to produce and the movements of the tongue and lips are small. Later the sounds become more complicated, such as 'bubbub' or raspberries and growls involving much finer movements of the lips, tongue or palate. It is hard to believe that a simple 'raspberry' sound is produced with very tight lips closed around the tongue and a strong force of air being pushed against it.

Vocal production now usually flourishes with a wide variety of sounds beginning to appear. Starting with one sound at a time, such as 'bu', the baby progresses to strings of sounds as in 'bubbubbub', eventually incorporating a variety of sounds within the one string that might sound like 'mumabubadugoo'. These sounds often seem to be produced for the baby's own enjoyment and it is common for parents to tell of 'little Jake lying in his cot for ages and ages just talking to himself'. Lips, tongue and

131

palate are all now given plenty of useful practice, with greater need for control as speed of use increases. However, as yet, no meaning or intent can be said to be involved.

The next step on the ladder of sound development usually involves linking sounds with actions or situations. Lip smacking or 'm' may begin as part of a mealtime routine, encouraged and modelled by carers. Similarly, sounds emerge such as 'br' when pushing a toy car or 'pa' during games involving smacking the bath water. The use of these sounds progresses to the point where infants are able to relate the sounds to specific actions or situations. At this stage they may begin to use their vocalizing more specifically to ask for something or to give information. For example, the child says 'br' and points out of doors to tell you there is the sound of a car outside, or smacks his lips together to indicate that he is hungry and wants something to eat.

During this time there is frequently a lot of 'sound practice', with infants babbling up to minutes at a time. These noises often sound very 'adult-like' and are beginning to include phonetic characteristics of the child's home language, such as English, Arabic or Cantonese. There are rises and falls in intonation reflecting those heard in the speech of carers. On picking up a toy telephone, a child may now consistently say 'eh-oh', linking the approximation of a sound she has often heard with an associated action. Singing nursery rhymes or songs now becomes a fun game, with imitated sounds being linked to familiar music and rhythms. Meaning behind the sounds is limited, but connections are being made between these sounds and their referents. More information on this stage of development is included in Chapter 7, in the discussion of the pre-verbal skills of performatives and protowords.

By the time children begin to attempt real words, they have generally been making a wide variety of sounds which, in English, include using the tongue:

- at the front of the mouth   t, d, n
- in the middle of the mouth   l
- at the back of the mouth   k
- with lips tightly sealed   p, b
- with lips lightly sealed   m
- with lips rounded   w.

At this stage, children will also have produced sounds requiring 'pops' of air as in 't', 'd', 'k', 'g', 'p', 'b' and attempted sounds requiring steady air flow such as 's', 'f' and 'sh'. Sounds requiring air to be directed through the nose rather than the mouth will also have been used, including m and n. Infants will have practised putting sounds at the beginning of syllables, such as 'bu', in the middle as in 'bubbu' and even at the end of syllables, as in 'bubbub'.

As infants experiment with sounds in words, some mistakes are expected. Examples of such frequently occurring 'errors' and common sound patterns associated with the production of early attempts are set out in Table 11.1.

Table 11.1 Examples of common sound patterns in early language

Common sound patterns	Examples
Omission of final consonants in words	'Book' ➔ 'boo', 'eat' ➔ 'ee';
Substitution of a similar sound type	'Sheep' ➔ 'see';
Substitution of earlier for later developing sounds	'Car' ➔ 'tar', 'rabbit' ➔ 'wabbit';
Lisp with tongue between the teeth	'Suck' ➔ 'thuck';
Consonant-blend reduction	'Snake' ➔ 'nake', 'climb' ➔ 'cimb';
Omission of unstressed syllables	'Blanket' ➔ 'bat';
Reduplication (complete or partial) of syllables	'Cuddle' ➔ 'kukoo';

Adapted from Rahmani (1987) and Shriberg and Kwiatkowski (1986).

The period in which errors such as those listed in Table 11.1 can be expected may last well into the period of early word combinations. A lisp, where the 's' is made with the tongue between the teeth, may be acceptable for a small child using single words. Such errors may last well into the period of first words and even simple sentences. Some children will still be making acceptable 'mistakes' for 's', such as 'think' for 'sink', even after they have begun to put in a marker to indicate plurals, as in 'carth' for 'cars'. Later on, when sentences have become more mature and vocabulary more varied, this will often have righted itself with a clear 's' being produced. Examples of the sounds you would expect to hear as children pass through the developmental stages proposed by Brown (1973) are set out in Table 11.2.

Table 11.2 Sounds expected in terms of expressive language structures (Brown's morphemes) and language stage

Sounds expected (approx. 75% accuracy word level)	Language structures; Brown's (1973) morphemes	Language stage (Brown, 1973)
h, ŋ (sing), p, m, w, b, n, a, t, y, k, g, ʒ (vision)	Present progressive -ing Plural s Possessive 's	2–3
f	Articles: a, the Regular past tense	4–5
Note: other sounds may be attempted, such as 's', but accuracy is not necessarily expected at this stage	Third person regular Third person irregular Uncontracted auxiliary (he is hopping) Contracted copula (he's tall) Contracted auxiliary (he's hopping)	

Source: Kilminster and Laird (1983); Brown, (1973).

Risk factors associated with the development of phonological skills

For the development of sounds to occur according to plan, muscles of the jaw, lips, tongue, palate and even the lungs need to be functioning reasonably well. Difficulty in coordinating movements or in holding muscles 'tight' may not make a noticeable difference during the production of the earlier sounds that require less effort to produce. However, a child's difficulties in these areas may become increasingly more apparent as the sounds to be produced become more complex. This may be of particular relevance for some children with problems in muscle coordination, such as those with Down syndrome (Stoel-Gammon, 1997).

Equally, for satisfactory progress to occur, children need to be able to hear sounds in their environment, as well as the sounds that they themselves make. Without adequate hearing, this environmental input and self-feedback is missed, with the possibility that sound-making may slow down or stop altogether. Some children are known to be at particular risk of a reduction in hearing due to fluid build-up in the middle ear (glue ear). This group includes children with Down syndrome (Rasore-Quantino, 1999), children in childcare settings (Froom and Culpepper, 1991), children whose parents smoke (Haggard, 1995) and children with enlarged adenoids (Silman and Silverman, 1991). The presence of sensorineural or 'nerve' hearing losses may also need to be investigated should sound development fail to progress.

General health of an infant may also play a part in sound development. An unwell, listless baby may not have developed the interest or even have the energy to produce sound, reserving its energy levels for the more important purpose of supporting life.

Encouraging the development of appropriate speech sounds

The types and amount of sound that children hear are important in developing their own sound output. As suggested in Chapter 4, talking to an infant is crucial, even at an early age, as it provides the building blocks for the child's future development of speech. The baby needs to hear speech sounds and intonation patterns. A baby left to play alone quietly in the cot for hours misses out on the language experiences needed for the production of sounds. On the other hand, if a baby is not very responsive to the noises the parents make, there is a risk that the parents will become discouraged and that sound play will lose its appeal. Perseverance by parents is recommended and will generally prove worthwhile.

It can be seen that, for young children, the production of speech sounds and the developments that can be expected at each stage are complicated. However, by monitoring what the child is doing, and providing appropriate sound models, you may be able to facilitate progress. If you are concerned about any aspect of the child's speech, follow your own intuition. Organize an assessment with an appropriate professional, such as a speech pathologist, as early as possible. In doing this, you may be able to minimize any long-term difficulties. In the meantime, the most important thing to remember is that most children learn skills more naturally through play and general life experience. It is not necessary for you to become a 'teacher' with structured lessons or tasks. Parents or carers talking to and generally interacting with their children throughout the day can provide plenty of opportunities for encouraging sound development.

Here are some suggestions for helping a child to develop effective sound-making skills:

- Remember that sound making should be enjoyable and interactive. The more fun an infant has listening to sounds and making sounds, the more sounds she will want to make. Getting a giggle from a parent by making a raspberry may certainly encourage many more raspberries to be blown. A father imitating his 'brilliant' child's use of his 'name' will certainly help to encourage that child to say it over and over. A cycle of mutual enjoyment will be the result.
- Remember that face-to-face contact between infant and parent allows the infant to see as well as hear sounds being made. Video-recordings of parents interacting with their babies (Trevarthen, 1979) have shown that infants will practise a face shape such as lip-rounding while carefully inspecting a parent's face during sound play. This will happen well before the children actually start to say the particular sound.
- Be aware that background noise such as television, radio and traffic can interfere with sounds being heard, particularly if the child has even a very mild (or intermittent) hearing loss. Should there be any risk the child is not hearing clearly, reduce background noise down as much as possible. Playing interactive games in a quiet room away from such noises may be a good idea. It gives the child the best chance of hearing all the sounds you are making. Children at risk of mild or intermittent hearing loss include those who have frequent colds, snore, or breathe through their mouths

Assessing early sounds

An outline of the stages of sound development in infancy is set out in Table 11.3. By listening to your infant's vocalizations, writing them down and checking against this chart, you will be able to determine a starting place to begin practising and encouraging sounds. For example, if the baby is starting to make a few different sounds, such as gurgles and squeals, you could make silly sounds by filling your cheeks with air and 'popping' them, or by making raspberries. Once the baby starts to eat solids, it is a good idea to try to leave the spoon in her mouth until she closes her lips on it. You can also begin to encourage the baby to drink from a cup. Both of these activities encourage development of muscle coordination and strength.

Table 11.3 Checklist for assessing and practising early sounds

Behaviour to check	Yes/No	Suggested activities for carers
1. Does the infant suck from a bottle or nipple? If yes:	Y/N	
i. Are the baby's lips sealed well?	Y/N	If you answer 'no' to any of these four questions, or if you have any concerns about feeding, talk to an appropriate professional, such as a nursery nurse, infant health sister, paediatrician, general practitioner or paediatric unit in a hospital.
ii. Is the baby sucking strongly?	Y/N	
iii. Does the baby take a long time to feed?	Y/N	
iv. Is the baby irritable during feeding?	Y/N	
2. Does the infant make a few sounds such as gurgles, varied cries and occasional squeaks?	Y/N	Make lots of 'small talk'. Say 'Hello, you've woken up. Time to get up, then. Off we go. Into your pram.' Have plenty of face-to-face time while you talk. Make silly sounds, sing-song noises; or make faces and noises to your baby, such as 'ooh-ooh', 'ah-ah' and raspberries, lip smacks, cheek pops. Have fun and try not to be discouraged by any lack of response.
3. Has the infant started solid foods?	Y/N	Leave the spoon in the baby's mouth until he closes on it. Encourage chewing and munching on a variety of toys, fingers then food. Some gagging on lumps is to be expected. Encourage food play to help build tolerance to different textures and sensations. Encourage drinking from a cup, even before the baby can reliably hold the cup. This encourages a more mature suck and swallow pattern, increasing co-ordination and strength. Ask for help if unsure.
4. Is the infant making more sounds, such as raspberries, growls, coughs, lip pops, tongue clicks or kisses.	Y/N	Try to copy the child's sounds. Remember to leave time for the child to 'talk back' to you. Encourage any sounds that you think the child could be making.

Table 11.3 Checklist for assessing and practising early sounds (contd.)

Behaviour to check	Yes/No	Suggested activities for carers
5. Is he or she making vowel sounds such as 'ah' and 'ooh' or consonants like 'b', 'm', 'n', 't' and 'd'.	Y/N	Encourage lip sounds and actions such as lip popping, lip smacking,' 'm', 'p', 'b', lip rounding and kissing. Encourage lips together when playing or sitting. Check that lips are closed when swallowing or eating from a spoon.
6. Is the infant mainly using tongue sounds like 'la-la', 't', 'd' and 'n'?	Y/N	Encourage tongue clicks, 'la-la', 't', 'd', 'n', sticking tongue out.
7. Is the infant mainly using lip sounds and actions?	Y/N	Encourage 'conversations'; talking to your child and leaving spaces for the baby to talk back to you.
8. Is the infant using long, complicated strings of sounds that seem like conversation?	Y/N	See Chapter 7 examples of sounds to link to particular actions or words. Chapter 8 has ideas to encourage development of real words.

Assessing early word skills

As with the suggestions made for checking an infant's early sounds, the easiest way to monitor early word production is by listing the child's spontaneous 'words'. Write the words down as they sound when the child produces them. You need this information in order to check that the child is able to make the sounds appropriate to his level of sound development.

Table 11.4 Earlier developing sounds and their position within the mouth

Common sound types	Position in the mouth		
	Front	Middle	Back
Pop	p, b	t, d	k, g
Flow	f	s, ʒ (vision)	h
Nasal	m	n, y	ŋ (sing)
Glide	w		

Look at your list of the child's words and identify the sounds that the are being used. You can use the checklist in Appendix E to record these sounds, or circle the sounds in Table 11.4. With this information, you will be able to answer the following questions:

• Does the child attempt a wide variety of sound types?
• Does the child attempt sounds in all positions within the mouth?
• Does the child use sounds at the:

– beginning of words?
– end of words?
– middle of words?
- If the child is not attempting a particular sound, will she use it in imitation?

If the child is spontaneously producing the types of sounds that are appropriate for his current language level as defined in Brown's morphemes (1973) (see Table 11.2) you will not need to give any extra practice. If the sounds are produced only in imitation, more opportunities to practise are needed. If the child does not produce the sounds at all, more specific help may be required.

Encouraging sounds that are not being used

If the child is not using some sounds, you need to provide opportunities to encourage the child to begin to attempt to practice producing them. When introducing such practice, remember the following points:

- Target only a small number of sounds at once as too many may cause confusion.
- Encourage the child to listen to the sounds when you say them. Saying them to the child, face-to-face, gives him an opportunity to hear the sound clearly and see how it is made.
- Use animal sounds ('I'm a creepy snake . . . s-s-s') or environmental noises ('Let's pop the bubbles in your drink . . . p-p-p') to help the child begin to attend to the sounds you are planning to practise (see Table 11.5).
- Link each sound to an object or picture and use the same signal whenever you practise that sound as in a ball 'b-', a car 'c-'.
- Let the child touch your face as you make the sound, allowing him to feel some of the sound's characteristics such as a puff of air ('p') or lips together ('m').
- Use gestures such as a fist popping open for 'p', 'b'. 't' or 'd' or a slow sweep of the hand for 'm' to give additional clues as to how the sound is made.

Reward the child's efforts with praise and a smile, a turn in a game, a sticker or any other treat you think the child will enjoy.

When you begin to practise making sounds with the child, start by getting him to:

- copy you:

  Adult: 'Pop the bubble, p'
  Child: 'p'.

- copy you after a delay:

  Adult: 'Pop the bubble. 'p. Now its your turn';
  Child: 'p'.

Table 11.5 Describing sounds to children

Sound	Description	Association
p	Put your lips together and pop (whisper)	p-p-p the 'boat sound' My Putt Putt Boat
b	Put your lips together and pop (loud sound)	b-b-b the 'bouncing ball sound' My Bouncing Ball
t	Put your tongue up behind your teeth and pop (whisper)	t-t-t the 'dripping tap sound' Mr Tap
d	Put your tongue up behind your teeth and pop (loud sound)	d-d-d the 'hammer sound' Mr Hammer
k	Put the back of your tongue up (pretend to cough or growl) Tilting the child's head slightly back or having them hold the front of their tongue down with a finger may help.	k-k-k the 'kookaburra sound' Mr Kookaburra
ch	Push your lips around and blow (whisper; a quick sound)	ch-ch-ch the 'train sound' Mr Train
m	Put your lips together and hum (feel the vibration by putting your finger on the side of your nose)	m-m-m the 'humming sound' Miss Humming
l	Put your tongue behind your top teeth (long sound)	la-la-la the 'singing sound' Miss Singing
h	Puff	h-h-h the 'panting dog sound' my panting dog
w	Move your lips around then back, from a kiss to a smile	w-w-w the 'stopping sound' Miss Stopping
g	Put the back of your tongue up (loud sound)	g-g-g the 'drinking sound' Mr Drinking
f	Bite your bottom lip and blow (whisper)	f-f-f the 'fly spray sound' Mr Flyspray
v	Bite your bottom lip and blow (loud sound)	v-v-v the 'plane sound' Mr Plane
s	Put your teeth together, smile and blow	s-s-s the 'snake sound' Mr Snake
z	Push your lips around and blow (loud sound)	z-z-z the 'bee sound' Mr bee
sh	Push your lips around and blow (whisper: long sound)	sh-sh-sh the 'be quiet sound' Miss Quiet
r	Put your tongue up to the top of the middle part of your mouth (sliding back from 'l' may help)	r-r-r the 'car starting sound' Mr Car

- say it on his own with a hint from you:

  Adult: 'Pop the bubble' (puts lips into 'p' position)
  Child: 'p'.

- say it on her own with *no* hints from you:

  Adult: 'Pop the bubble'
  Child: 'p'.

Once the child has mastered a sound on its own, you can try to *combine it with a vowel* as in 'pa', 'pe', 'po' *using repetitive sequences* of the same sound such as 'p' and then progressing to *using the sound in simple words* such as 'pat', 'pet', 'pot', 'pin'. Remember that the words the child uses first are most likely to be those that are of high interest and also the easiest to say. Try to avoid introducing words that *you* think are important. Follow the child's interests.

Suggestions for practising sounds in words

As previously noted, it is acceptable for some 'mistakes' to be made in words in the early stages of learning to talk. However, having chosen which 'mistakes' to target for change, start with the sounds that are in only one position in a word, such as the beginning or end as in 'car', 'cow', or 'up', 'cap'. Practising the sound in all beginning, middle and end positions can be confusing for the child. You may decide to practise more than one sound at a time, but it is a good idea to focus on no more than three target sounds at the same time. When you begin to practise new sounds, remember to:

- Accept the child's attempts to say a word. Repeat the target word correctly, slightly emphasizing the incorrect sound. For example:

  Child: 'dere du'
  Adult: 'yes, there is a duck. Duck. The duck says quack, quack. Duck'

- Increase the frequency that the child hears the sounds in words by reading through a list of words that use the 'target sound' each day. You can pair each word on the list with a picture. For example, if the target sound is 'k' in initial word position, use:

  Cow
  Cat
  Car
  Comb
  King

- Use the words in fun situations to encourage the child to practise without even recognizing she is doing so. For example, stock the bath with toys that use the required sound to increase opportunities for the child to attempt to say the word and hear it modelled correctly. Other routine times during the day that lend themselves to this type of 'stocking' include:

- mealtimes
- in the sandpit
- story time (make up your own stories if you cannot find any to suit)
- dressing
- shopping

- Move your hands to show how sounds are used or not used in words. For example, if the child is missing the beginning sound in a one-syllable word like 'ball'; put your closed fists side-by-side at eye level. Open each in turn to represent the first and second parts of the word, as in:

'b'   'all'
open one fist   open second fist

By opening only one hand at a time, you can describe which part is actually being missed. For example:

(b)-   'all'
keep fist closed   open fist

Say: 'I could hear the last part. I wonder what happened to the 'b' at the beginning?'

'b'   '-all'
open one fist   open second fist

- Look through books or magazines together to find pictures of things that have the sound you want to practise. Model and describe the word. Encourage the child to say the word, rewarding and describing the practice sound as necessary. Cut out the pictures and paste them in a scrapbook or put them in a 'treasure box' for later practice.
- At the supermarket, find as many items as possible that include the practice sound. Encourage the child to say the word as the items go in the shopping trolley and again, when they are unpacked. Naming things can also be played at mealtimes, bath-time and during any joint activity during the day.
- Hide several pictures or objects that have your practice sound in them. The child has to find an object, put it in a 'sound spot' such as a box or basket and name it. Again, praise, modelling and description are required from the adult.
- Picture lotto or picture/object matching games can also increase the opportunities to hear and practise the target sounds in words.

Recognizing different sounds and how sounds work in words

The ability to recognize subtle differences between two sounds, an important skill needed for the accurate reproduction of sounds in words and the development of word comprehension, may not be automatic for all children. Some children commonly mistake 'Where's your nose?' for 'Where's your toes?', suggesting that they have misheard the question. For such children, *difficulties in auditory discrimination* make learning to understand the words they hear very difficult. Modelling pairs of words and demonstrating the differences between them can help to build the level of children's awareness of sounds in words and hopefully alleviate some of these difficulties. Some word pairs that could be used in a 'Give me . . . ' game with pictures include:

nose	toes
horse	sauce
dolly	lolly
red	bread
clothes	close

Although this chapter has focused on the child *making* sounds, it is also wise to understand that the *recognition* of sounds and how they work in words (phonological awareness) are important elements in the skills needed for early literacy. A child's ability to recognize syllables in words as in 'do – lly', the two elements in single syllable words such as 'd – oor' and the single sounds in words such as 'p-e-n' are skills used in decoding written words. Children need to begin to develop phonemic awareness during the early years of childhood. Focusing on speech perception and production can be beneficial in developing these skills. This means that the work done to encourage children's intelligibility through demonstration of words and language may well have a secondary beneficial effect in supporting early literacy skills. Information on issues raised in this chapter can be found in Buckley (2001), Buckley and Bird (2001) and Cupples (2001).

Summary

This chapter has introduced the path of sound making from birth to the use of words and early sentences. This is not always an easy progression. Sound-making is complicated by 'mistakes' which may be stress-inducing for carers but which are actually regarded as acceptable. By monitoring areas of concern, it is possible to determine the significance of the sounds being used by a child relative to his or her developing language and, if necessary, provide opportunities to maximize the child's sound skills. This will further encourage growth towards effective communication.

Chapter 12
Augmentative and alternative forms of communication as stepping stones to speech

Earlier chapters have demonstrated that learning to talk is one of the most complex tasks that children master in their early years. Even before they are able to use words and sentences, most children begin to use a variety of ritualized sounds and gestures to communicate their wants, likes and dislikes. Gradually they learn the combinations of sounds and words that form the spoken component of their language.

For some children, the process of learning to talk is particularly long and difficult. Those who experience a range of specific intellectual, physical or neurological disabilities may have problems developing the skills necessary to communicate verbally with others. Children who suffer frequent ear infections may have difficulty at critical times in hearing clearly what is said to them, and as a result are slow to develop speech. A few have motor planning problems or oral or verbal dyspraxia which leads to difficulty in organizing the speech muscles to produce specific sounds or sound combinations. These children begin to develop expressive language skills but are unable to produce words clearly enough for a listener to understand. Others, including children with autism and related neurological disorders and those with relatively poor auditory attention and processing skills, may experience difficulty in developing meaningful social communication skills using speech. Other forms of communication such as the use of natural gestures, facial expressions, pointing to pictures, manual signs, or, for some, voice output communications aids to complement or, if necessary replace speech, may assist such children to acquire early communication skills.

In many day-to-day conversations with children, adults use gestures to emphasize what is being said. For example, Mummy says 'get the book; it's somewhere over there' while pointing in the general direction of the missing item, describes the giant as 'huge', with arms reaching high, or picks up the ball as she says 'let's play ball'. At snack-time she holds out the cheese and the sultana jar as she asks 'do you want cheese or sultanas' or holds out the carton as she says 'look, we've got orange juice today'. At the milk bar she asks 'Which one do you want?' as she points to the picture display of the different ice creams available. The visual information from these gestures, objects and pictures adds meaning to the spoken words. These situations also occur when young children begin to convey their own messages. For example, Denny looks up at Daddy after completing his puzzle, smiles and claps his hands. The message is: 'I've finished, aren't I clever'. Kate sits in her trolley and wriggles backwards and forwards while looking at Daddy. It's clear to him that she wants to be pushed. Sometimes objects are used. Claire tugs Granny's skirt and pulls her to the fridge as she hands Granny her empty bottle: the message here is 'I want something to drink'. Mark is sitting on Mummy's knee as she reads a magazine. When he sees a picture of a red car, he slides down and runs to get his red car and shows it to her; his message is 'I've got a red car too' or 'This is a red car like mine'. Often a sound is included in these communicative acts which will continue to be used until the child is able to produce recognizable words to convey meaning.

Visual communication symbols are about us everywhere. Children soon learn to recognize the 'stop' sign and that the green light means 'go'. They recognize the white marks on the road or the pedestrian crossing symbol when Mum says 'We need to cross the road'. Most children instantly recognize the McDonald's big M and are quick to request a visit there when they see it. At the store, Ravi picks up a copy of his favourite cartoon video and hands it to his mother. Marie is quick to see a preferred toy in the store catalogue, pointing to it as she hands the book to her mother. Once children are able to talk, they continue to refer to objects and pictures to reinforce their meaning.

This chapter is concerned with the use of non-verbal means of communication, often referred to as augmentative and alternative means of communication (AAC), the signs and picture communication aids that are used to supplement the speech of children experiencing difficulties in expressing and/or understanding spoken language. A brief description of the different types of AAC is given. The reasons why different forms of AAC can be used to help some children to learn to talk are considered. Suggestions are made for deciding which children may benefit from learning to use signing or picture communication aids, vocabulary choice, the context in which such procedures are used and other issues involved in their implementation.

Why introduce a non-verbal augmentative communication system?

There are many reasons why the introduction of non-verbal means of communication can be a positive step in helping children to develop meaningful communication and, hopefully, meaningful speech. Children who have developed clear intentional communication but are not yet using consistent sounds or words may be experiencing delays or difficulties in phonological development or in making the transition to using vocal forms of communication. The use of gestures and other informal physical or visual aids to communication is a natural part of everyday language. It adds to the message that is given, allowing what is being talked about to be seen as well as heard. Congruent use both of spoken words and of their visual representation to help a child to learn initial vocabulary is likely to be more effective than the use of spoken words alone. Children remember the speech sounds associated with a particular entity, such as 'drink', but also remember the visual image of the object, picture or hand movement that is consistently paired with the word. Some children, particularly those with severe learning disabilities, perform cognitive tasks more effectively when presented with material in a visual or concrete mode, rather than a purely auditory mode. The likelihood of recall is enhanced when information is accessed through more than one sense. In this way the augmentation of speech through the use of manual signs and other aids supports language learning and enhances the cognitive level at which the child is able to function.

There is general agreement (Bloomberg and Johnson, 1991; Beukleman and Mirenda, 1998; Dice, 1994; von Tetzchner and Martinsen, 2000; Koul, Schlosser and Sancibrian, 2001) that the introduction of visual forms of communication may be helpful for some children in the early stages of language acquisition. In particular, it may assist children who are at risk of, or are already, experiencing problems in understanding and using language. Gesture appears to play an important part in the early stages of communication development by providing a visual prompt to assist in the comprehension of messages (Martinsen and Smith, 1989; Acredolo and Goodwyn, 1990; Erting and Volterra, 1990). The use of gesture declines as children are able to speak more clearly (Goldin-Meadow and Morford, 1990). Wilcox and Shannon (1998) suggest that until the brain has reached a stage of maturation compatible with verbal representations, it might be more effective to assist the child's communication development through enhancement of non-verbal skills. Signing can supplement, and in some cases replace, other more primitive forms of communication. Children with verbal dyspraxia, or deficits in auditory perception can augment or replace the use of speech with signing or pointing to photographs or picture symbols to communicate. Ryan (1996) has presented evidence of the facilitative effect of the use of signing on the social and emotional development of a young child with Down syndrome.

Mirenda (2001), Ogletree and Harn (2001) and Koul, Schlosser and Sancibrian (2001) have all presented evidence supporting the use of visual speech symbols such as photographs or pictures for children with autism who generally have relatively strong visual-spatial abilities. Stiebel (1999) assisted the parents of several children with autism to communicate spontaneously by using a variety of three-dimensional objects and photographs in relevant daily routines. Children with restricted or impaired movement skills, as in Angelman syndrome and cerebral palsy, have been able to achieve effective functional communication through the use of simple signs or three dimensional objects, pictures, picture symbols or voice-operated communication aids (VOCAs) (Stiebel, 1999; Dicarlo and Banajee, 2000).

Experience of the authors in working with young children with a range of delays in developing communication and developmental disabilities suggests that an AAC can relieve stress not only on the child but also on family and carers. For carers, it removes the guesswork in understanding a child's behaviour. The facilitative effect on the child's communication of using a mutually recognized and acceptable alternative form of communication has, in turn, a positive effect on the relationship between the child and other children and carers in out-of-home group situations.

At a more practical level, adults often speak too fast for children to hear and process the message being sent. In this situation, comprehension is enhanced if speech is supplemented with gestures or other aids that reinforce the message being conveyed. When using a gesture, sign or other visual aid in conjunction with speech it is common for the speaker to slow down, either to recall a specific sign or find the appropriate picture, to add emphasis, or to ensure that the listener has seen and attended to the whole message. The pause allows more time for the information being sent to be received and understood. It also helps to reduce any overload that may occur when well-intentioned carers talk too much when interacting with a child. By using a visual prompt, such as a picture or sign, eye contact can be encouraged with those children for whom lack of attention or poor eye contact is an additional part of their communication difficulty. For example, some signs involve making rapid finger movements near the face, as in the Auslan or Makaton sign for 'there' (see Figure 12.2). Such movements often seem to encourage the child to turn to look at the speaker rather than attend to just the spoken word alone. If a child is looking away from a speaker's face, using the hands to gain attention and draw gaze back into the face-to-face position encourages the eye contact necessary for effective interaction. A physical prompt to respond can be given by shaping the child's hand to gesture or sign towards a picture or object of interest.

Types of AAC systems

AAC systems can be classified into two main groups:

- *unaided systems*, which involve the use of idiosyncratic gestures and signing, and
- *aided systems*, which require the use of some equipment or manual communication aids such as objects (real or miniature), photographs,

picture symbols or pictographs, communications cards, boards and books, or electronic communication aids such as calling and scanning devices and voice output communication aids (VOCAs).

The form of AAC to be introduced will depend on a number of factors including the nature of the child's difficulties, the current stage of the child's communication development and the ability of the child's family and carers to implement the agreed system.

- *Gestures* are the simplest form of AAC and are used by most people in everyday communication. Some children experiencing communication difficulties develop their own gestures, or adapt those used by others. In the early stages of language development these may be sufficient to get the communication process under way. However, they have the disadvantage of being idiosyncratic and may be understood only by a small number of the child's potential communication partners.
- *Signing* using an established signing system such as American Sign Language (ASL), Auslan, British Sign Language (BSL) or Makaton can increase the potential for the child to communicate with a much wider group of partners. No equipment is needed and it can be used to develop both receptive and expressive language skills. Vocabulary can be expanded as needed. Evidence suggests that once children begin to develop effective verbal communication they drop the use of signs. However, signing requires reasonable control of hand and arm function, visual and memory skills, and recognition that a hand sign conveys a certain message. Communication partners must also learn to sign.
- *Visual-aided systems* have proved to be particularly useful for children with fine motor and other muscular difficulties, or relatively poor auditory perception and processing abilities. Choice of the form of visual-aided AAC will depend on the stage of communication development of the child as well as physical and cognitive development.
- *Objects, or parts of objects* such as toys or food packets, provide excellent visual information about the activities or events available. They are often useful for children in the very early stages of developing intentional communication (see Chapter 10) and for those with more severe physical limitations or with intellectual delays and disabilities. However, they can be bulky and difficult to transport and the range of functions for which they can be used is limited.
- *Photographs*, particularly those that depict objects and activities that are familiar to the child, can be used to encourage early communication in young children. Photographs of familiar objects and people offer similar advantages to objects, are usually highly motivating, are easy to produce and relatively easy to transport; for example, mounted in a small folder or album. However, as the child begins to interact with a wider range of objects and people in a range of different environments, it may be more practical to introduce the use of picture

symbols. Computer-generated picture symbols such as Boardmaker and Picture Communication Symbols (PCS) have the advantage of being reproducible in a variety of forms, either as pictures placed on individual cards or in a book, or even in electronically operated displays. As more generalized pictures, they can be used to convey the child's message in a wider range of communicative contexts.

- *Electronic devices* such as calling and scanning devices and VOCAs have been shown to be helpful for some non-verbal children with developmental disabilities They can be rewarding for the children, as they are not easily ignored. However, they can be expensive, may have limited accessibility and range of application and may require specialized programming and technical support.

Who could benefit from AAC?

Children who might benefit from the introduction of AAC as a supplement to speech include:

- those who are known to be at risk of significant delays or difficulties in understanding or using spoken language. This group can include children with Down syndrome and other syndromes with known craniofacial abnormalities and narrow eustachian tubes; young children with mild developmental delays who suffer from frequent colds which can depress hearing levels for periods of time, and those with general developmental delays and moderate to severe learning difficulties
- children who continue to demonstrate marked difficulties in producing understandable speech despite previous involvement in other language development services or programmes. For these children AAC may become a more permanent mode of communication.

The initial aim of AAC is to provide a greater opportunity for children to understand spoken language. For these children, AAC is used as a 'scaffold' during the period when a child with delayed language begins to communicate more effectively. Therefore, although some consideration should be given to the child's fine motor control when deciding whether or not to introduce signs, this may not initially be a major factor to consider. When a child begins to use signs, an approximation of the desired hand movement is generally acceptable, provided it conveys the required message. Fine tuning of movements can be done later. However, when children seem to be physically unable to produce even simple hand movements, an alternative system should be considered. This might be an aided system involving the use of:

- real objects, photographs, drawings, picture symbols or pictographs
- small line drawings that represent specific concepts such as the boardmaker with COMPIC (COMPIC, 1989)

- Picture Communication Symbols (PCS) (Johnson, King and Sloan, 1993)
- Rebus (Clark, Davies and Woodcock, 1974)
- Bliss symbols (McNaughton, 1975)
- communication boards (see Jones and Cregan, 1986; Bloomberg and Johnson, 1991)
- electronic (voice-output) systems.

When should an AAC be introduced?

Parents and carers begin to teach spoken language to their children from the moment they are born, gurgling, singing, talking and playing with them. Language teaching occurs all the time, with parents frequently unaware of the impact of these activities on children's development. Once an infant or child has been identified as being at risk of significant disruption in language growth, additional methods of communication can be introduced by parents and other carers. These will supplement the child's speech and maximize the impact of the messages the child is receiving and sending. Sometimes this process can begin soon after birth. In other cases, speech is not augmented until much later, when the child has not begun to talk as expected. By introducing the chosen system as early as possible, parents maximize the possibility of the child understanding and using the system communicatively. The process for assisting children to learn to use signs or other visual systems will be considered later in this chapter.

Which AAC system should be used?

A number of issues should be considered when selecting an AAC system for a child. You will need to take into account the child's particular needs and skills. For example:

- Is the system likely to be temporary, as a support until the child's oral language skills become adequate? Is its main purpose to encourage comprehension? Is it likely to become the child's main method of communication in the long or short term?
- Is the child physically capable of using the proposed system? Does the child have adequate control of fine motor movements to make hand signs? If signs or symbols are being considered, are they sufficiently iconic to be understood by relative strangers? Is the system portable? Can it be used in a wide variety of settings? Can it be easily learned by the child? Is there a financial consideration?
- How likely is it that those people in direct contact with the child will learn and use the system? What, if any, system is used in the preschool, school or other setting or situation in which the child is likely to be involved?

You may decide to use a combination of AAC systems, or a Total Communication (TC) approach (Gibbs and Springer, 1995), particularly if you are working in a group situation with children with a range of needs. In an inclusive classroom with both typically developing children and those with additional needs, the typically developing children soon learn the additional forms of communication and provide excellent support and peer modelling for those with additional needs. By fostering the use of a combination of systems, all children are encouraged to communicate, each using the most effective method in terms of their own needs. A small number of children with more severe physical or intellectual disabilities may need to use calling or voice-operated systems to initiate interaction. Whichever system, or combination of systems, you decide to use, you should monitor its implementation to ensure that the needs of the child continue to be met. In particular, you should check that the vocabulary continues to be adequate for the child's expressive and receptive needs. In addition, other communication partners need to be informed of any changes that are made. You will also need to continue to monitor whether or not an additional or alternative system should be included in the child's communication options.

Choosing initial vocabulary for augmentative communication

Each child is an individual, with his or her own particular needs and interests, and these should be kept in mind when you select an initial vocabulary for a child. Children's main interests are often associated with food and favourite toys and activities, so if Joshua's favourite food is cheese, you can begin by using a picture or the sign for cheese. If the child loves to listen to tape-recorded songs, introduce the sign or picture for 'music'. The sign or picture for 'bath' may be used to signal bathtime. At this stage, the names of objects and routine activities are often the most frequently used.

For common meanings for which there are no concrete referents, such as 'gone', 'more' and 'finished' or 'no more', signs are often most useful. These signs are often easily recognizable. Even children with poor sight or poor fine motor control can learn to use variants on basic signs, particularly those that involve some body contact or gross movement of the hand. Examples of such iconic signs include two fingers touching the mouth for 'food' and a cupped hand tipped towards the mouth for 'drink' (see examples of frequently used Makaton signs, Figure 12.1). Other simple commands or requests such as 'give', 'look', 'sit' or 'point' can also be introduced to assist the child's understanding of what she is being asked to do.

You should also consider the frequency with which the item is used in the child's everyday life. If the child goes to regular therapy or educational

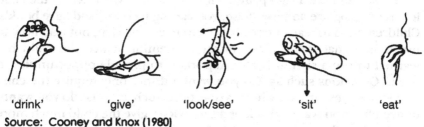

'drink'   'give'   'look/see'   'sit'   'eat'

Source: Cooney and Knox (1980)

Figure 12.1 Examples of single commands

programmes, you may wish to start using signs or pictures to represent the people he will see or the activities that he will participate in. If you are working in a group situation where there is a regular timetable or routine, signs or pictures for key activities such as snack-time and story-time can often be of help to a child who has difficulty with moving from one activity to another.

How is AAC introduced?

You can initially introduce signs or pictures as an integral part of your natural communication with the child. How this is done will depend on the child's needs and the type of system chosen.

Signs

If you decide to use signs, look for a system that uses clear, easy to make, iconic signs. If the child already has a number of clear natural or idiosyncratic gestures, it is best to accept these and use a sign from a recognized signing system for new words. You will find it easiest to introduce them as a part of your natural language. This will involve always pairing a gesture or sign with the spoken word.

- Whenever you speak to the child, use the gesture or sign concurrently with your words. To start off, it is particularly important that the child learns to link the sign with the object or activity that it represents. To ensure this, you will need to make sure that the child sees the sign and experiences the associated referent simultaneously or as close together as possible. For example, if you are offering a drink, make sure you have the cup or juice carton either in your other hand or close by as you sign and say 'juice' or 'drink'. If you are going out in the car, say and sign 'car' as you reach the car.
- Once the child learns the meaning of the sign, you will be able to use it without the actual object or activity present. You do not need to pair every word in a sentence with a sign, only the key words. For example, for the sentence 'let's go in the car', you can start by signing only 'car'. 'Give me

the book' can have a sign paired with 'book' or 'give'. Later, as the child learns to recognize and use these, you can sign 'go car' and 'give book'.

- Children need to learn not only how to make the sign, but also how to use it to signal their communicative intention. Once the child has learned to use a sign, it is also important to provide opportunities to use it. Questions such as 'Do you want a drink? only require the child to respond 'yes' or 'no', whereas questions such as 'What do you want?' or even 'Do you want a drink or a sandwich?' give the child much more scope to use those signs that have been learned.

- Sometimes, learning by imitation is not enough. You may need to begin by physically assisting the child. To do this, you should take the child's hand and help make the required sign while saying the word at the same time. This process is called 'shaping'. Such assistance may be particularly useful for children with severe difficulties and delays because it also involves their tactile sense (sense of touch) and will help to avoid repeated failure. Once the child is able to produce the sign, a physical prompt such as lightly touching the child's hand may be sufficient until the child can use the sign without help. Children respond positively to the experience of achieving success, even though the actual attempt by the child to use a sign is assisted. It is crucial to encourage the child to look at both the speaker and the sign as it is being made, so try to keep your hands as close as possible to your face while signing as a way of encouraging face-to-face interaction. As has already been suggested, this also encourages eye contact and improved attention to the speaker.

The more people who are involved with introducing signs to a child and the more fun that is had doing it, the greater the chance that the child will develop the use of signs as a supplement to his or her growing language skills. When a child begins to use signs, it is a good idea to compile a 'dictionary' or 'my words' book to help other people recognize what the child is telling them. This should involve drawings or photographs of the signs that the child uses, and descriptions of how they are made. Put the signs together with a picture of the object or activity. A good example of this is found in *A Picture Dictionary of Australasian Signs for young Children* (Hondow and Watchman, 1990). Any idiosyncratic variation used by the child should also be noted. Those interacting with the child can refer to this book to check on current vocabulary, any variations used by the child and how the signs are made. This is particularly useful when the child's signs are not clear. From the child's point of view, the most important point is that messages are being received and understood.

Remember, when you begin to introduce signs to a child:

- Before signing a word, try to ensure that the child is watching you.
- Always say and sign the word at the same time.
- Encourage the child to sign as you would encourage speech. For example, 'tell me . . . '.

- Introduce only one or two new signs at a time.
- Before expecting the child to use a sign, make sure you give plenty of opportunities for him or her to learn what it means.
- Expect the child to sign just as you would expect speech.
- Accept any approximation of a sign at first, but as the child becomes more capable, expect and encourage the clearest sign that the child is able to produce.

To enable the child to have lots of practice, you can introduce appropriate signs into favourite action songs such as 'Old Macdonald had a Farm', 'Miss Polly had a Dolly' and 'Hi, Good Morning'. Videos of signed nursery rhymes and favourite children's songs are available, for example *Makaton Nursery Rhymes for Australian Children* (Variety Club of Australia). Use signs as you look together at picture books and family or group photo albums. Signs can be used with most of the games suggested for helping a child to learn first words (see Chapter 8).

If you decide to use a manual sign system, some useful sources of information include Sternberg (1994), Brennan, Colville, and Lawson (1984), Walker and Cooney (1984), Miles (1988), Johnson (1989), Hondow and Watchman (1990), and Jeanes, Reynolds and Coleman (1993).

Picture communication

Pictures, including photographs and picture symbols, are often introduced to assist:

- children who are not yet using sounds but are able to get their message across by pointing
- those with good visual skills and poor auditory and attending skills
- those with motor difficulties who know what they want to say but are having difficulty producing accurately sounds or sound combinations.

If you decide to use pictures, you may wish to start of with clear photographs of the child's own familiar possessions and for very young children and those with significant delays in receptive language and cognitive development, pictures of activities involving familiar people. Children with good receptive language skills can be introduced straight away to picture systems such as COMPIC (1989) or PCS (Johnson, King and Sloan (1993). These are available as computer software and are often used by speech and language pathologists, early childhood programmes and schools attended by children with developmental delays and disabilities. They have the advantage of including a large range of different everyday actions, activities, places and feelings as well as familiar objects.

If you are introducing picture communication to a young child:

- Before you start, collect photos or pictures of things in the child's regular environment; for example food, toys, clothes, bed, bath. For durability, cover the pictures with clear plastic adhesive film, or laminate them.

- Choose two or three things the child wants but is unable to ask for using words, for example 'juice', 'ball'.
- When giving the food or playing with the toy, point to the picture as you introduce the object. For example, to introduce 'juice' put the picture alongside the juice carton and say 'juice'. Pour a little into the cup. Then wait for the child to indicate that he wants more. Encourage the child to point to or touch the picture for you to pour some more. If necessary, physically assist the child to touch the picture. Similarly, pair the ball with the picture of a ball as you introduce a game with balls.
- When the child uses a picture to identify objects or services, give her a choice between two pictures. For example, ask if the child wants milk or juice. Point to the picture of each in turn as you ask 'Do you want milk or juice?'
- Leave the pictures in a place where the child knows the food or toy is kept, for example pictures of food on the refrigerator or cupboard and toys and pictures of toys on the toy box.
- If you have spare copies of pictures, use a small ring binder or notebook to make an album of words for food or clothes that are familiar to the child and that can be taken to preschool or daycare.

Once the child understands the meaning of each picture and can use them to request or give information about what he or she is doing, you can start to use them in combination to make sentences. For example, the child can point to the picture to request 'I want' plus the food, toy or activity as in 'I want a banana'. By using a felt board and a simple fastener on a smooth surface, you can even make up a visual daily or weekly timetable which you can use to assist the child with remembering routine activities and to introduce variations to a routine. This can be helpful for children who have difficulty managing their behaviour as they not only hear but also see what is available or required.

If using pictures or picture symbols to assist children with making choices or following as sequence of activities, a red diagonal cross can be used to indicate that an activity is over or no longer available. The cross should be large enough to cover the picture or symbol (see Figure 12.2) and the child told that it is now time to finish playing with that object or activity. The child will soon understand the meaning of the cross. Similarly, a red cross can be attached to objects or fixtures, such as cupboard doors, electrical switches or television controls to indicate that they are not to be touched.

If you are working in a group, a visual timetable is useful for letting everyone know the daily programme. Children who have difficulties remembering the routines can be encouraged to check on the board. To help with making choices and task completion, children can be encouraged to choose an activity picture from the board and 'post' it in the 'finished'

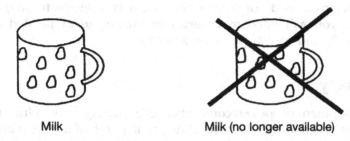

Figure 12.2 Example of a symbol 'no longer available'.

box once they have completed the activity and before choosing another. Even children who can talk will often refer to the 'daily programme' to find out what activities are available before making a choice. For children from a different home-language background, the picture remains constant even though the actual words are different. Even after children start to speak, they are able to refer back to the pictures in times of uncertainty or stress.

Children with limited communication and motor abilities can learn to use a picture board to indicate basic needs such as food or drink, 'more', or to respond 'yes' or 'no' using pictures attached to a cardboard or wooden board.

As with signing, taking the time to ensure that the child understands what a picture represents and how to use it is important. Adults need to be consistent in their use of the pictures to encourage the children to use them.

Other aided communication systems

For young children with limited cognitive abilities, plastic fruit or actual food packages attached to a large piece of cardboard may help with making choices. Their use is generally limited to a narrow range of choices and applications, but they can be useful in reducing stress and frustration for both carer and the child.

Calling and other electronic communication devices are not generally used with very young children but they have been shown to be useful in helping children with severe disabilities to initiate communication and make limited choices in early intervention programmes.

Combining systems or total communication

By using a total communication approach, children are provided with opportunities to develop those forms of communication that work best for them. Total communication (TC) is particularly useful for helping children to express early semantic relationships using single and two-word combinations plus sign utterances. As children progress beyond this stage, their preference for speech or sign provides a practical indication of the preferred mode of communication. If you decide to adopt a TC approach, you will need to ensure that the resources needed by the child's family and relevant staff are available.

Summary

The development of spoken comprehensible language is the ultimate goal for almost all children. The use of different forms of augmentative and alternative communication systems tailored to their individual needs is one way to help achieve more effective communication for children experiencing difficulties in the early stages of language development. Evidence suggests that both signs and picture communication systems may facilitate and will certainly not interfere with the child's acquisition of language and, in particular, intelligible speech. Either singly or in combination, they can help children to experience the benefits and fun of communication. They should be accepted as a useful tool for children who are struggling to acquire effective language skills.

Chapter 13
Working with children whose home language is other than English

Helping children with communication difficulties whose home language is different from the major national language presents a double dilemma for the teacher or therapist. First, there is the question of adequate assessment of the stage of the child's communication development and whether the child is experiencing difficulties in:

- the process of developing communication
- learning the language of the new linguistic and social context.

A decision about which language the family and professionals should use in assisting the child must be made; the parent's first language, or the language of the community in which they now live.

Whatever language is being learned, it appears that its acquisition is governed by a combination of maturational and environmental factors, with the environment providing a particular language system as well as the context for its acquisition (see Chapter 2). There are similarities in the stages that all children pass through in the acquisition of their first language (Bloom, 1970; Brown, 1973; Halliday, 1975; Bates et al., 1979; Warren and Yoder, 1998; Wilcox and Shannon, 1998). Moreover, carers in all cultures use language to interact with their children and support and guide their acquisition of language, even though the values placed on different adult strategies for facilitating the development of language may vary (Chiocca, 1998; Wilcox and Shannon, 1998). As has previously been suggested, learning to talk, even in the child's first language, is an extremely complex task.

Children who are already experiencing difficulty in learning a first language at home are faced with an even greater task when placed in a new language context such as a childcare centre or preschool. Research on language development in children from bilingual backgrounds suggests that the more skilled they are in their home language, the better able they are to learn a second language (Ramsey, 1987). Furthermore, the importance of the social context in which language is acquired is recognized, with the quality of adult language input contributing significantly to the child's early communication development (Salinger, 1988; Duncan, 1989; Deuchar and Quay, 2000; see also Chapter 4). Makin, Campbell and Jones Diaz (1995) have pointed out the importance of recognizing and preserving children's cultural and linguistic diversity, while at the same time assisting them to become effective communicators in English, the language that they encounter once they enter a playgroup, preschool or other early childhood programme. Makin et al. support the use of the child's home language and have documented the benefits of providing early instruction in the home language within non-home settings. Makin (1992) demonstrated the social and motivational benefits to children in both formal and informal early childhood settings when periods of home-language support are provided on a regular basis. This form of support may be particularly desirable for children who are experiencing delays in the development of their home language (Duncan, 1989) and whose parents are not highly proficient in the community language (Toppelberg, Snow and Tager-Flusberg, 1999). They further suggest, however, that the advisability of maintaining the home language should be balanced against the benefits to the child of learning the language of the wider community, coupled with any limitations in the child's ability to learn two languages.

It is important to remember that children who are having difficulty developing communication skills in their first language will inevitably experience difficulties in acquiring a second language. This has significant implications for professionals who are using a language other than the child's home language when assisting children with language delays and disabilities (Toppelberg, Snow and Tager-Flusberg, 1999). Many children entering a non-familiar language environment for the first time have to become used to not only the new social context but also to a different linguistic context. For some, this can result in a silent period (Krashen, 1982; Roseberry-McKibbin, 1994; Clarke, 1999) as they attempt to master the different linguistic aspects of the second language environment. Their apparent difficulties in developing communication skills may be related more to their need to adjust to a new linguistic and cultural environment than to difficulties in learning to talk. Provided that their pragmatic, phonological and semantic skills are developing normally, most children will soon adjust to the new linguistic environment as they learn the equivalent words in English (Deuchar and Quay, 2000).

When deciding to assist a child from a different language background, it is important, first, to consider the extent to which the child is competent in both the home language and the major community language (Santos de Barons and Barona, 1991; Chiocca, 1998). Firstborn or only children may have had very little exposure to the major community language. On the other hand, children who have family members including older siblings who are linguistically competent in the major community language may have developed skills in both languages. Similarly, those who have had regular exposure to the major community language through preschool or other forms of out-of-home care may also be competent in both languages.

As children develop early language skills, whatever language is used, efforts need to be made to provide assessment and learning conditions that encourage meaningful interaction with significant people in activities that are developmentally and culturally appropriate.

Assessment

As has previously been suggested, careful collaborative gathering of information and setting of targets and strategies with family members is likely to lead to more positive outcomes for all participants. Activities chosen should be both developmentally and culturally appropriate. How, then, should the assessment of communication development in children from linguistically and culturally different backgrounds be approached?

The importance of assessment in routine settings involving activities that are meaningful to the child has already been discussed (see Chapter 5). However, the extent to which you are able to access some of the child's regular settings may be limited, depending on the child's family, the availability of personnel who are familiar with the child's linguistic and cultural background and culturally appropriate resources. Whether or not you decide to use English to carry out assessment of the child's communication skills, you will need to have information on the child's competence in the home language.

When qualified, competent speakers of the child's home language are available, they can undertake assessment tasks with the child as well as gaining information on competency in the home language from the family. What form this assessment takes will depend, in part, on the availability of culturally appropriate resources. As far as possible, the child's family should be involved in the assessment process, which should be undertaken in the child's dominant language. However, when the parents do not speak English well and you are not familiar with the family's home language, you will need to consider other options. For example:

- Qualified interpreters can assist in obtaining reports from parents and carers on the children's language competence at home and in regular care settings.
- Interpreters can assist in the administration of both structured and unstructured assessment tasks, including observation of the child's communication strategies and competencies.
- When trained interpreters are not available, other members of the family circle may be able to provide assistance as interpreters. However, this is not recommended unless suggested by the child's parents, as it may not always be culturally appropriate.
- If the child attends an early childhood programme, a carer in the child's nursery school, preschool or childcare centre who speaks the child's home language may be able to assist with the assessment, including the gathering of observational data.

- If possible, the person who is to take primary responsibility for assisting the child in developing new language skills outside the home should be present during any assessments and, if appropriate, take part in the assessment process. This will enable the carer to observe the child's inter-action strategies during assessment and will also provide useful information for later programming to support and assist the child.

When no support from interpreters or family members competent in both languages is available, you will need to rely on your own observation of the child (Duncan, 1989; Mills, 1993). Reliable information can be obtained about the child's understanding of basic concepts by using appropriate everyday materials and careful observation over a range of sit-uations, including play and familiar routines.

Warren and Yoder (1998) suggest that early communicative intentions are probably cultural universals and are unlikely to vary significantly between different societies. Although there may be differences in the combination of sounds used by children from different language back-grounds, the activities in which they are engaged when they make these sounds provide clues to their meaning or significance. For example, while eating or feeding a baby doll, an English-speaking child may accompany the action with 'yum yum' whereas a Cantonese-speaking child may say 'oum'; putting a doll to bed, a French-speaking child may use the performative sound 'do-do' but an English-speaking child says 'ni-ni'. Whatever the sound combination used by the child, the parent or inter-preter will soon confirm whether the sound is specific to the activity and whether it is regularly used in their language community.

For children who are already using words, you may need to ask some-body familiar with the child's home language – a parent, teacher or classroom aide – to translate the child's words for you. Any sound com-bination regularly used in a specific context should be checked with a person who is familiar with the child's home language. For example, a French-speaking child may say 'la' to point out an object of interest or try to direct an adult's or child's attention. A French speaker will confirm that the child is saying 'there' to indicate the existence of a familiar object or to direct the adult's or child's attention to a particular event. A child whose family speaks Arabic at home may regularly say 'ana' when approaching other children or an adult. An Arabic speaker may indicate that the child is saying 'me'. Further observation and discussion with the child's family may confirm that the child is using the word 'me' to indicate a wish to play with a toy or to request permission to join in an activity.

A tape-recorder or video-recorder may be useful in observing a child in a naturally occurring or structured assessment situation. However, make sure you have the family's permission to record the session and to view the taped material, as this may not be acceptable to some families. You can then use the tape to assess and to discuss with the parents how to interpret what is happening. Even if their command of the major community language is limited, parents are usually happy to assist, if asked, by indicating whether the child's utterances include performative sounds used in their language, real words or phrases. It is also important not to neglect the child's use of gesture to communicate. Communicative gestures vary between languages and cultures, so it is important to check the meaning of any gestures used regularly with a person who is familiar with the child's language and cultural background. As with monolingual children, it is important to make every effort to obtain accurate and relevant information from a variety of sources.

Implementing a programme

Once you have completed your assessment, you will be able to provide useful opportunities for learning, provided you adhere to a few simple procedures. For example:

- Respect the families' linguistic differences and cultural preferences in choosing strategies to support the child's language learning, both in choice of play materials, approach to play and involvement in family routines.
- When working with families, allow the parents to choose which language they will use at home. Some families will prefer to use the major community language used by most other children at the preschool or nursery centre. This can have benefits in meeting the child's long-term communication needs. Whichever language you decide to use, it is important to choose learning targets that best meet the communicative needs of the child.
- If you are working in a preschool, nursery school or daycare centre, unless you have staff and children familiar with the child's home language, you will probably use the language dominant in the centre for most communication with the child. Signs and, particularly, other visual forms of communication such as pictures may also help, as the sign or picture remains the same regardless of the language used. The suggestions in Chapter 12 may assist you in choosing appropriate augmentative strategies and materials.
- You must ensure that the family is aware of the language you are using. They also need to know any relevant vocabulary, as well as the forms of language, including any signs, gestures or other augmentative materials or strategies being used for giving information and instructions. If necessary, seek the assistance of a competent speaker of the family's language to pass this information on to them.
- If there is a member of staff in your centre who speaks the child's home language, this may be the most appropriate person to act as the primary carer for the child.
- Involvement of other children with the same home language in routine activities and play may also help the child. A linguistically competent

child from the same language background may be happy to become a 'buddy' to the child who is experiencing difficulty, helping the child to negotiate the unfamiliar language environment. The suggestions in Chapter 14 for using routine situations and play when working with groups of children are also appropriate when implementing language objectives for children who do not speak English at home.

- For children at the preverbal stage, although there are variations in performative sounds and communicative gestures used by people from different language backgrounds, many are similar and actual functional play with objects, such as pretending to drink, rocking a baby, pushing a car and stacking blocks, is not culturally dependent.

- If you suspect that the child is having difficulties in language acquisition, it may be useful to initiate the use of agreed augmentative or alternative forms of communication such as signs or pictures even before the child starts using words. Chapter 12 on augmentative communication sets out further suggestions on when and how to begin such a programme.

- For those who are using early words, or who are ready to practise them, it may be helpful to follow an agreed or standard signing system, and to give the opportunity to make choices using pictures, in conjunction with both the home and major community language. The sign or picture will stay the same, regardless of the language used, providing a consistent referent and a bridge between the two languages.

Remember, whatever the stage of the child's language acquisition, the use of frequently occurring routines, developmentally appropriate strategies and materials, and language-rich activities including action songs, rhymes and language-based games and activities, will help the child in learning to operate successfully in the new language environment.

Summary

This chapter has considered some of the issues that arise when teachers, therapists and others encounter a child whose home language is not English and who is experiencing difficulties in developing communication skills. In helping such a child, you should remember that the basic processes underlying the development of early communication are universal. However, you will need to be aware of differences in the linguistic contexts of the child's home background and use strategies that are culturally sensitive. You will also need to ensure that these strategies take account of the child's long-term needs and are introduced and modelled in such a way that parents and carers feel both involved and comfortable with the choice of language and procedures that you are implementing.

Chapter 14
Working with children in groups

Many of the ideas suggested in this book for encouraging the development of early language skills have focused on individual children and their specific needs. Strategies have been described for pinpointing a child's current language level; selecting appropriate objectives such as specific actions, gestures, sounds or words; choosing activities and materials that will give opportunities to practise the new skills; and checking on progress.

Situations are described in earlier chapters for implementing effective strategies for helping children involved settings where an adult spends time alone with a child working through selected activities. All these tasks can be carried out in a variety of contexts. A parent may help a child at home, during special playtimes or routine daily activities with siblings. However, for many reasons, parents are not always able to help their children learn new skills. Some children spend much of the day in a preschool or daycare centre. Others learn more quickly when another adult helps them – therapist, teacher or nursery aide, rather than a parent. Teachers and others carers working in the early childhood field are sometimes the first to recognize that a child is experiencing difficulties in learning to talk. For some children, the playgroup, preschool or nursery school is an ideal setting for learning and practising new language skills. Many children respond to situations where they can watch, imitate and learn from their peers. Even children who are developing new skills in one-to-one situations benefit from opportunities to practise them in group settings such as an early childhood centre where they have regular contact with other children and adults. This chapter is concerned with the strategies that can be used by teachers, therapists and others to implement language objectives for an individual child in a context that involves groups of children.

There are a number of advantages associated with the implementation of language objectives for a child in contexts that involve groups of children.

- *Generalization of emerging language skills*: Early childhood pro-grammes usually provide a variety of activities for the child to participate in. When helping a child to learn new language skills, it is important to provide opportunities for the child to practise the skills in a variety of situations. This ensures generalization of the skill to con-texts other than that in which it is first learned.
- *Opportunities for imitation of appropriate language models*: Other chil-dren in the group model appropriate language for the child to imitate.
- *Development of pragmatic skills:* Participation in social situations pro-vides children with opportunities in which to learn to communicate intentionally in a naturally occurring social context.
- *Opportunities for practising newly acquired language skills*: Children can begin to use emerging language skills during interaction with peers and other adults.

When helping children with language difficulties within a group context, it is very important that your goals for each child have been identified. You can ensure that the children have opportunities to hear appropriate lan-guage modelled by other children as well as adults, and to use those actions, signs, sounds or words that have been selected for practice. You can also take steps to see that other adults who have contact with the children are aware of the language objectives that are being targeted, and can help in their implementation.

In this chapter we shall consider three types of group situations that can be used for encouraging and practising language and communication:

- structured or planned group activities
- unstructured or informal group play
- informal and naturally occurring routines.

Many opportunities for encouraging language occur naturally during the day as part of the familiar sequence of events that fill the timetable of a busy early childhood programme. Think about the routines that are repeated each day, as the children arrive, put away their bags and coats, greet a staff member and settle into play. Later, there are the relatively fixed times for eating, toileting, hand washing, sleeping, small-group activities with a teacher or carer and, at the end of the day, going home. During the day, children frequently spend time playing in either large and small formal or informal groups with construction toys, with dolls in 'home corner', in the sandpit, or painting, writing, running, jumping, singing and listening to music or a story.

Strategies for helping children develop the pragmatic or social aspect of language are discussed in Chapter 10. Group settings such as early childhood programmes are ideal places for children to develop and prac-tise intentional communication as they learn to ask for food and drink and to negotiate their way through the range of activities that they encounter with other children in both small and large groups.

Structured or planned group activities

Some of the activities that occur regularly in most early childhood settings are relatively structured, with accepted procedures that children need to learn to follow. Newly enrolled children must learn how to behave in these activities. They need to learn the pattern of the daily routines so that they can behave as expected, in terms of both their actions and language. For example, during story time they must sit quietly, not wriggle, listen, watch the teacher and the book, and be ready to answer any questions that are asked. Look for language objectives that can be practised during these routine activities.

Unstructured or informal group play

Other situations such as outside play and dressing up or imaginative play are less structured, giving the children greater freedom to act spontaneously and follow their own interests. The children need to learn how to act in these situations and this is often achieved by watching the other children and imitating their actions and words. You should also be aware that some of the children who are having difficulty in communicating with their peers and other adults in the centre may benefit from the introduction of alternative and augmentative communication systems such as signs, photos or pictures to support their communicative attempts (see Chapter 12). If any children have learned to use signs or consistent gestures you will need to find out which words have been learned and how the signs or gestures are performed.

Scripts for informal and naturally occurring routines

The idea of 'scripts' was introduced in Chapter 3 as a way of explaining the way in which children's concepts or mental schema for familiar events develop. Children make sense of the daily events of their lives by learning the 'scripts', or the actions and language associated with these events. If you are working in an early childhood programme and need to identify specific language objectives for particular children in the group, one option is to identify the language components of the scripts associated with the more structured activities in your programme. You can then plan ways to encourage the children to acquire these language skills. You should begin by observing the children and analysing the daily programme to identify the routines and associated scripts followed by the children at different times of the day. These situations are good contexts for teaching language. For example, the actions and words used in greeting and farewell routines and during mealtimes (e.g. 'more', 'no', 'juice') can be practised here. Other words associated with art, craft, painting, and time with the teacher also provide opportunities for practising script-based communication.

Implementing a language programme

Starting off

Before beginning to assist a child with delays or difficulties in developing language, you will need to decide on a starting point. If another professional has not formally assessed the child's language level, use your own informal observations of the child's current language level and knowledge of the sequence of the development of children's language. You can use the assessment activities suggested in Part 2 (Chapters 6–10) and record the results of this assessment in the summary assessment sheets provided in Appendix B.

Next, you need to select some simple targets or goals for the child that you and your colleagues can implement and monitor while the child is at the centre. If you are working in a preschool, nursery school or childcare setting, the language targets can be included in your regular observation and planning cycle. These cycles usually cover a 4–6 week period and this is an ideal time-frame to allow for the child to achieve success in the current target. Take care to select targets that can be practised in situations that you and the child are likely to encounter frequently.

Make sure that other people in the group setting are aware of the objectives and strategies that you have chosen for the child. Some people like to keep a written record of these objectives and of the child's progress and other staff can contribute to this record with additional information on the child's achievements. Maintenance of such records is sometimes a requirement of government funding authorities, particularly where additional funds are provided to assist children with delays or disabilities who are attending an early childhood centre. Displaying the children's targets and strategies in a simple format where they can be seen and referred to as necessary by all staff in the room will help to keep everyone aware of what they can do to assist individual children. Staff may then record when they observe instances of the targeted communication behaviour. Record forms that can be used for this purpose are included in Appendix C. However, it is important not to allow such recording to interfere with or distract you from achieving your primary objective, which is helping particular children learn to communicate better.

Much of the learning that occurs in early childhood settings is achieved during daily routines and naturally recurring activities when children choose what to do or play with, interact with other children and adults, and move from one activity to another (transitions). Opportunities to practise targeted language goals can be found at many different times during the day.

Practising language objectives

Some of the best opportunities for learning language in a group occur when the children are engaged in structured or regularly occurring group activities. Much of the language used in these situations involves familiar 'scripts' and even children who are not yet talking know what to do when they greet and leave other people, either smiling and waving (gesturing) or saying 'hi' or 'bye'. At birthday parties, they know that everyone sings 'Happy Birthday to You'. As they are given food or a present, they know that they say 'ta' or 'thank you'. If they are unfamiliar with what is said and when, they soon learn from hearing what the other children do and say. More competent speakers in a group provide excellent models for less proficient children to copy. So look for activities where the child has opportunities to use language in routine situations and where other children are involved, and encourage the child to join in. 'Home corner' or the dramatic play area, or even a table with a telephone, provide excellent opportunities for encouraging children to use familiar scripts, so try to include these when planning opportunities to practice your language objectives.

Morning snack-time is an example of a daily routine that can provide children with opportunities to practise language skills. Each child in the group can be asked 'What do you want?' and then encouraged to answer by saying, signing or pointing to a picture to indicate, for example, that they want a drink or some fruit. Visual supports such as the actual fruit or drink can be shown to assist them in their choice. You can vary your expectations for each child according to their language level. For example, initially you may expect a child only to look at your face before being given something to eat or drink. Gradually, this expectation can be changed as the child learns to say 'milk' or 'juice' or point to the item of choice, when prompted. Use the binary choice or the C-I-C strategy (see Chapter 8) to provide a model of the words or signs to be used. Eventually, the child will learn to ask by using sentences such as 'Can I have a drink, please?' or 'May I have an apple?'.

Table 14.1 shows a sequence of objectives that you can use for children who are learning to ask for their juice and fruit. It gives you some idea of the changes in learning to ask and can be adapted for use in any situation

Table 14.1 Suggested sequence of objectives for learning to ask

Adult: 'Do you want a drink?'	Child looks at adult
Adult: 'Lorie say/tell me . . .'	Child uses sound and/or sign or points to picture e.g. 'j' or 'm' to obtain a drink
Adult uses C-I-C strategy or binary choice	Child says and/or signs name, e.g. 'juice' or 'milk'
	Child names or signs, e.g. 'juice'
	Child extends request to two-word sentence, e.g. 'want juice' or 'Lorie juice'
	Child extends to three-word sentence, e.g. 'I want juice'
	Child uses request form, e.g. 'Can I have juice'
	Child uses question form, 'May I have juice please?'

during the day when the child may want something. Remember to prompt the children at each stage, asking first 'What do you want?', pausing to give the child time to respond and then, if there is no reply, using a binary choice such as 'Do you want juice or apple?' or the C-I-C strategy with 'What do you want? 'Say (or tell me) milk.', then, 'what do you want?'

With regular practice, children will gradually improve from simply looking, to using simple gestures, sounds or single words, to asking properly by using complete sentences.

A similar procedure can be used in other formal and informal individual and group situations. For example:

- asking for toys or activities during informal playtimes
- asking for assistance with personal activities, for example taking off and putting on shoes, washing hands
- asking for help at any time – 'help' and 'help me' are very useful words for a child who is having difficulty learning to ask for assistance

Informal and formal group activities that include recurring patterns of behaviour provide some of the best opportunities for learning. For example:

- While learning to match objects to pictures, each child can be encouraged to say or sign something at an appropriate level while engaged in the task. A child who is not yet talking may make an appropriate sound, such as 'br'mm', to accompany the car that is being matched to a picture. A more competent child might be encouraged to label the car or use a simple sentence such as 'Daddy's car' or 'Daddy's got a red car' as part of the game.
- In a group activity with building blocks, one child might be encouraged to say 'er-er' while moving a heavy block into place, while another might be encouraged to comment that 'it's heavy', talk about where it is going or what they are building, as in 'it's a boat'.
- Other situations where this approach can be used include water and sand areas, dough table, joint craft or painting activities, in fact any activity where children are engaged in a shared task that is supervised by an adult who can give encouragement to ask for objects or assistance.
- Some of the best opportunities for practising language occur during the telling and retelling of familiar stories, particularly where a story involves the repetitive use of language. These situations are useful because the children do not have to think of something to say. They need only to remember their part in a story, or listen to what the other children are saying. Traditional 'scripted' stories, such as *The Three Bears*, Lynley Dodd's *Hairy Maclary* or Pat Hutchins' stories, which use frequent repetition of key words or phrases, give the children the opportunity to say together repeated parts such as 'Who's been sleeping in my bed?' Some children may be able to say only a single word or part of the phrase, but they have the satisfaction of joining in. Simple puppets can be useful in assisting children with their parts during story telling.

- Favourite songs and nursery rhymes with frequent repetitions of words and phrases can also be used to practice language objectives. Children can sing together 'e-i-e-i-o' or take turns to name the animals or their sounds in 'Old Macdonald Had a Farm'. If signs are used when an animal is named, children who are signing can actively join in the activity with the other children.

Structured or planned group activities

Children often learn useful speech from listening to other children modelling appropriate words and you can take advantage of this in many situations. For example:

- Singing and circle games such as 'Ring-a-Ring-a-Rosy', 'Here We Go Round the Mulberry Bush', 'Hokey Pokey' and 'Duck, Duck, Goose' provide children with clear actions to perform, such as dancing in a circle, falling down, turning or running around as they sing or say the words. All these games give children clear instructions about what to do and, more importantly, what to say.
- Regular greeting and goodbye songs with the whole group provide similar opportunities. They are useful situations for encouraging children who lack confidence in participating in group activities.
- Games using the surprise bag described in Chapter 7 can also be used as a planned group activity. You might like to use different food and eating items (banana, cup, spoon), clothing and personal items (hat, shoe, brush), household equipment (doll's house chair, table, bed), toys (ball, car), animals (dog, cat, cow) or even objects that start with the same sound (ball, book, bear). Depending on their level of language, each child can make a sound, say or sign the name, or talk about the colour, function, size or texture of the chosen object.
- Board games that can be played at a table or on the floor can be used to practise language. A lotto game using pictures of objects, animals or events (shopping, a party, bath-time) and cards with sets of matching pictures allow children to learn by imitating their more competent peers. A more competent child or adult can act as 'banker' naming each card as it is picked up from the pile, or children can take turns to pick up and name the card or to ask 'Who has . . . ?' A more able child, or an adult, can model such language for a child who is difficult to understand. All children in the game have the opportunity to participate, to indicate 'My turn', 'Me', 'I do' or perhaps to label the cards using sounds, words or signs. The child who is learning to talk has repeated opportunities to hear and use useful words and sentences. Picture dominoes and 'snap' games can be used in a similar way.

An advantage of using group activities, as well as turn-taking and the frequent repetition of useful words and phrases, is the opportunity they provide for children to talk according to their current capability while still being part of the group. The games themselves should be enjoyable and continue for each child for only as long as he or she is interested. In addition, children learn that talking is worthwhile because speech makes something happen in the game.

Unstructured or informal group play

As noted in Chapter 3, some of the most valuable situations for helping children to acquire language are associated with those activities and contexts that allow children to explore and use materials and equipment freely, to pretend and to simply interact informally with other children and adults. Examples of these situations include:

- *materials and equipment:* playing with blocks, Lego, puzzles, dough, paints, sand and water
- *pretend games:* doll's corner, dressing up, tea parties, cooking in the sandpit, going shopping
- *informal games:* chasing, hide and seek, climbing together on A frames and jumping and bouncing together on the crash mat.

Children can be encouraged to practise emerging language skills during these informal games by an adult commenting, prompting and modelling targeted sounds, actions and words such as 'on', 'in', 'roll', 'cut', 'splash' 'up', 'down', 'pour tea', 'that's nice', 'oh oh, fall down', 'your turn', 'me too'. If possible, encourage more competent children to allow the child to join in such games so that they have conversational partners who can help them to extend their language. You may need to join in the game during the early stages, but try to withdraw as soon as the children are able to continue the activity without support. Just sitting near a group of children who are playing or doing the same activities near each other will encourage them to communicate with you. Other children will hear what you say and you can encourage them, if necessary, to communicate with others nearby.

Remember that in an early childhood setting, children are most likely to talk with other children during:

- informal games
- gross motor and simple social play: swings, trikes, rough-and-tumble, 'horsing around'
- group routines such as morning snack
- non-playful social interaction when there is no task involved
- pretend play

(Source: Sylva, Roy and Painter, 1980, p. 87)

They are most likely to talk to an adult during:

- activities involving genuine attempts at reading, writing and counting
- non-playful social interaction such as borrowing, giving help, teasing or being cuddled
- structured materials such as puzzles and dominoes
- art when under the direction of an adult

(Source: Sylva, Roy and Painter, 1980, p. 88).

Advantages of working in a group

A major limitation to the effectiveness of language development programmes implemented while working with children in one-to-one situations concerns generalization. Children need opportunities to use newly acquired skills in other settings, outside the classroom or clinic where the initial learning has taken place. One of the most important functions of children's informal games is to provide opportunities for children to generalize new skills; to begin to practise the social use of language by communicating spontaneously in natural settings, with peers and other adults. Indeed, it can be argued that, in order to be confident that the child's language activities have been successful, you need to observe the child using newly acquired skills in informal games with peers, or in contexts other than those in which they were acquired. Early childhood and other group settings provide ideal contexts for this to happen.

Finally, it is worth noting that, for most children, language objectives are achieved most quickly if they are shared between home and the child's playgroup, preschool or other early childhood programme. The selection of language objectives, their implementation and the monitoring of progress can be shared across home and other settings, with parents and teachers, therapists or other interested adults contributing to the child's progress.

Summary

When planning a language programme for a child, remember that new language skills can be practised in structured or semi-structured one-to-one activities (Chapters 6–10). However, if you have the opportunity to help a child in a context that involves groups of children, you should remember that your goals can be implemented in:

- informal and naturally occurring routines
- structured or planned group activities
- unstructured or informal group play.

The most effective learning will take place when opportunities for talking occur in many situations during the day. So make sure that you take advantage of all possible occasions for practising new language skills. The most important thing to remember is that you expect from children only what they are capable of, at their particular level of development.

Chapter 15
Working with families

Earlier chapters have considered how language develops and how a child who is experiencing, or is at risk of, delays in language development can be encouraged by a familiar adult (teacher, therapist, nursery nurse or other carer) to acquire the skills needed for effective communication. In any activity designed to help with children's development in the early years the family must be central to the process. This is particularly so in the development of early language and communication skills. Mothers and other primary carers support the development of those skills which combine to bring about the growth of early language and communication. The earliest interactions between mother and child set the pattern for the social as well as language development of the child. Interactions with significant people in their environment help to shape the communicative initiations and responses of the child long before the first word is spoken. At the same time, the linguistic and social context of the family has a significant effect on the family's ability to assist and support their children.

Children experiencing, or at risk of, delays in language development will inevitably need enhanced support from their families if they are to develop effective communication skills. However, this need for additional support must be balanced against the abilities, needs and wants of the family as a whole. Indeed, Dunst, Trivette and Deal (1988) stress the need to consider the context of the family in any attempt to assist a child experiencing developmental difficulties. In addition, there is continuing recognition of the importance of providing assistance to children any with additional needs in a collaborative mode (McCollum, 1999; Turnbull et al., 1999).

Setting up a programme for a child

Once it has been agreed that a child will benefit from additional assistance, consideration can be given to who will provide such help, what form it will take, how it will be provided, and for how long. It is essential that the family is actively involved, or that there is at least one member of the family who will take a central role in supporting the child. This is essential if the programme is to lead to lasting benefits for both child and the family. The process involved can be both formal and informal. Many professionals find it useful to start by developing an individual family service plan (IFSP). Programmes that are subject to government funding often have this as a central requirement for the provision of funds. Even if you and the family are not governed by such constraints, an agreed written plan, including a starting point, together with short-term targets and strategies, provides an excellent framework for ensuring that everyone involved with the child can know how to assist the child. These plans do not have to be elaborate. A simply written statement of achievable goals and strategies is often of most value to busy parents and is more likely to lead to successful outcomes for the family as well as the child. However, to arrive at this point, the family, and particularly the child's primary carers, need to feel confident about their role in the child's programme and their ability to do what is required.

What then, are the essential components of a language programme if the process is to be of benefit to the child while, at the same time, minimizing disruption to the functioning of the family as a whole?

Starting off

Experience has taught us that the first key to successful collaboration between parents and professionals is to consider the association as a partnership. As in all partnerships, each member brings their own attributes to the shared venture. The professionals provide the knowledge and skills required to facilitate the child's language development, but it is the family that supports the child's attempts to negotiate the wider environment using emerging language skills. To allow the family to make informed choices and to ensure that a cooperative partnership will develop, the following are essential:

- See the family as central to the whole process of their child's learning to talk.
- Listen to the concerns and wishes of the family.
- Accept and take into account their wishes and concerns at all times.
- Find out what they know about their child's difficulties in acquiring language and possible reasons for these problems.
- Get to know who is the child's primary carer and supporter within the family.
- Find out the family's current priorities for the child.
- Observe and take into account family interaction styles.
- Ask how they would like you to help them with their child's language development.
- Allow them to choose the people, both within and outside the family, whom they will involve in the programme.

Remember that while you may have expertise in issues associated with language development, it is the parents and family who are the experts on the child and how their family system operates. They are the ones who know how much they can contribute to the child's programme, how much they want to know, and how fully they want to be involved in the teaching process. You may find the parent inventory in Appendix F useful in finding answers to these questions during your initial contact with the family. However, it is important to remember that, if the relationship between you and the family is to provide optimum support for the child, you will need to review the association constantly and be sensitive to any changes in the family perspective.

Initial assessment

Formal assessment tools such as developmental assessments and language assessments will provide valuable information on the child's current level of language development. This information can also be used to identify appropriate starting points for intervention. However, this is only a small part of the picture. In an assessment situation, for a variety of reasons, children do not always demonstrate their true abilities. To be successful, you and the parents, together with the whole family, need to agree on where to start. Within the assessment process, involving the parents and other family members or carers acceptable to the parents, provides a wider perspective on the child's language competencies. Observation of the child in a familiar environment is the optimum assessment situation, but whether or not this is done, much can be learned about the child's current level of language development, parental and family strengths, understanding and interaction styles through observation and discussion during the assessment process. This is often a significant factor in achieving successful outcomes for the child. Involvement of parents in the assessment process allows you to discuss what you observe about both child and parent behaviour and also fosters an open, positive relationship between you and the family

Setting up a child's programme

Once initial assessments are complete – and this may take more than one session – discuss the results with the family to identify a realistic 'starting off' point. Rather that setting formal aims and goals for the child, it is often better to state the objectives that you hope to achieve in the form of *desirable outcomes* for the child. For example, it might be suggested that Mithra's mother and grandmother could 'encourage greater use of single words during normal daily activities, when looking at books and while playing with Mithra'. Several appropriate situations may be identified through discussion and agreement reached on the range of words that can be encouraged in these situations and the amount of time that will be allowed for reaching this goal. The actual choice of objectives and a time frame is then left to the family. This approach ensures that neither family nor child feels pressure to 'perform' in a set way. Ensure that they have the necessary materials and information to assist them in implementing the planned goals and in sharing these agreed strategies with other family members.

General practical and written information can be shared with the family during the early stages of setting up a child's programme. This can include:

- practical demonstrations of strategies that the family might attempt to use
- written information on the process and levels of early language development and the adult's role in children's language development
- suggestions for appropriate adult language
- ways to encourage play.

Copies of written information that can be used in this way are included in Appendix F.

Encourage the parents to tell you about their child and to share family concerns as they work to enhance the child's communication skills. Being open and encouraging two-way information-sharing will encourage the family to take on ownership of their child's programme, and boost their confidence in their own ability to provide appropriate on-going support for the child.

Be prepared to change or vary suggestions or ideas that may not be working for the family. Any strategy that they are not comfortable with is less likely to be followed through, or at best only poorly implemented, and this will lead to a less successful outcome for both family and child.

Some strategies for helping family members to become effective communication supporters and partners with the child include:

- *role play or role exchange* in a turn-taking setting, such as tea party, bathing a doll, or games with blocks, cars and balls
- *modification of adult language models* to a level commensurate with the child's, aiming to achieve a discrepancy sufficiently challenging to ensure the child's progress towards the next level (see instruction for taking a language sample, Appendix A)
- *review of parental use of appropriate language* including commenting, modelling, prompting, binary choice, expansion, extension, and use of home rules.

Regular sessions, on a mutually agreed time schedule, also give families opportunities to raise and discuss other relevant issues, such as:

- where to find out more information relevant to their child's needs
- where and how to find toys and other materials to use in helping the child

- the process of language acquisition and parenting issues
- further education for the parents about their child's disability and needs
- ways to increase their effectiveness as supporters of their child
- stress management techniques
- how to make contact with other parents and support groups.

Be prepared for progress to be slow, particularly in the earlier levels of language development and when the child has associated developmental delays or disabilities that may affect the language development process. Consider with the family whether the use of alternative and augmentative forms of communication, such as signing or pictures, might help the family and the child to communicate better with each other. Ideas on how to introduce an alternative or augmentative form of communication are set out in Chapter 12.

Experience has shown that, although it is helpful, it is not necessary for the teacher or other professional to speak the same language as the family in order to help them and their child achieve success. Openness to their linguistic and cultural context will more than make up for lack of a common language. If the child's family is from a language background other than English, you may find useful information to assist you and the family in Chapter 13.

Links with other agencies

When children attend a preschool, daycare centre or any other early childhood intervention or therapy programme, contact and cooperation with staff there is recommended. This ensures that targets and strategies being developed in the language programme are compatible with those from other services. It is often possible to agree, in consultation with the family, on common targets and strategies. As well as reducing possible stress and confusion for the child, it can considerably ease the load on already busy parents. The links should be made only after reaching agreement with the family on who will make the initial contact with other agencies and who will be responsible for continuing contact. On a practical note, a clear written record of any contact with other agencies will enhance the benefits of making these links.

Evaluation of programme impact

Regular, on-going evaluation of the impact of the programme will help everyone involved to maintain its effectiveness. Frequent formal evaluation of progress is neither necessary nor recommended. Observational and anecdotal evidence, as recommended for initial assessment, are highly effective, particularly once a positive partnership with the family has developed. If you decide or are required to provide formal evidence of progress, involve the family in the process as much as possible.

Moving on

As with any early childhood intervention programme, the time comes for the child and family to move on. If the child is moving on to another programme, contact and discussions, involving the family, before the change is made will ensure that the transition is smooth and trouble-free for both the child and the family. If, for some reason there are limits to the time that you can be involved with the family, make sure that they are aware of this from the beginning and ensure that they continue to be aware of the short- or fixed-term nature of the programme. If your initial and continuing aim has been to help the family to develop appropriate knowledge and skills to help their child, moving on will be a positive experience for everyone involved.

Summary

An individualized approach to assisting each family, along with sensitivity to different family structures, needs, and management styles will enable parents to develop their skills in such a way that they are able to take a more informed role in encouraging their child's language development. Putting the family at the centre of the process, sharing with them your knowledge and skills and taking into account their own needs, operating styles and systems, will ensure that they are able to take a more active and informed role in encouraging their children's language development. This, in turn, will ensure that the best possible outcomes are achieved for both the child and the family.

References

Acredolo L, Goodwyn S (1990) Sign language among hearing infants: The spontaneous development of symbolic gestures. In: Volterra V, Erting CJ (eds), From Gesture to Language in Hearing and Deaf Children. New York: Springer-Verlag, pp. 68–78.

Ainsworth MDS, Blahar M, Waters E, Wall S (1978) Patterns of Attachment. Hillsdale, NJ: Erlbaum.

American Psychiatric Association (1994) Diagnostic and Statistical Manual of Mental Disorders, 4th edn. Washington, DC: American Psychiatric Association.

Andersen ES, Dunlea A, Kekelis L (1984) Blind children's language: resolving some differences. Journal of Child Language 11, 645–64.

Austin JL (1962) How to Do Things with Words. Oxford: Clarendon Press.

Barrett M (1995) Early lexical development. In: Fletcher P, MacWhinney B (eds), The Handbook of Child Language. Oxford: Blackwell, pp. 362–392.

Barton M, Tomasello M (1991) Joint attention and conversation in mother–infant–sibling triads. Child Development 62, 517–529.

Barton M, Tomasello M (1994) The rest of the family: The role of fathers and siblings in early language development. In: Gallaway C Richards BJ (eds), Input and Interaction in Language Acquisition. Cambridge: Cambridge University Press, pp. 109–134.

Bates E (1976) Language and Context: The Acquisition of Pragmatics. New York: Academic Press.

Bates E, Snyder L (1987) The cognitive hypothesis in language development. In: Uzgiris IC, Hunt JMcV (eds), Infant Performance and Experience: New Findings with the Ordinal Scales. Urbana, Ill: University of Illinois Press, pp. 168–204.

Bates E, Bretherton I, Snyder L (1988) From First Words to Grammar: Individual Differences and Dissociable Mechanisms. Cambridge: Cambridge University Press.

Bates E, Dale PS, Thal D (1995) Individual Differences and their Implications for Theories of Language Development. In: Fletcher P, MacWhinney B (eds), The Handbook of Child Language. Oxford: Blackwell, pp. 96–51.

Bates E, O'Connell B, Shore C (1987) Language and communication in infancy In: Osofsky JD (ed.), Handbook of Infant Development, 2nd ed. New York: Wiley, pp. 149–203.

Bates E, Benigni L, Bretherton I, Camaioni L, Volterra V (1979) The Emergence of Symbols: Cognition and Communication in Infancy. New York: Academic Press.

179

Beilin H (1978) Inducing conservation through training. In: Steiner G (ed), Psychology of the 20th Century. Vol 7, Piaget and Beyond. Zurich: Kindler, pp. 260–289.

Benedict H (1979) Early lexical development: comprehension and production. Journal of Child Language 6, 183–200.

Bertoncini J (1998) Initial capacities for speech processing: Infants' attention to prosodic cues to segmentation. In: Simion F, Butterworth G (eds), The Development of Sensory Motor and Cognitive Capacities in Early Infancy: From Perception to Cognition. Hove, East Sussex: Psychology Press, pp. 161–170.

Beukleman D, Mirenda P (1998) Augmentative and Alternative Communication: Management of Severe Communication Disorders in Children and Adults, 2nd ed. Baltimore, Md: Brookes.

Bloom BS (1964) Stability and Change in Human Characteristics. New York: Wiley.

Bloom L (1970) Language Development: Form and Function in Emerging Grammars. Cambridge, Mass: MIT Press.

Bloomberg K, Johnson H (1991) Communication Without Speech: A Guide for Parents and Teachers. Hawthorne, Vic: Australian Council for Educational Research.

Bochner S (1986) Development in the vocalisation of handicapped infants in a hospital setting Australian and New Zealand Journal of Developmental Disabilities 12, 55–63.

Bochner S, Price P, Jones J (1997) Child Language Development: Learning to Talk. London: Whurr.

Bochner S, Price P, Salamon L (1988) Learning to Talk: A Programme for Helping Language-Delayed Children Acquire Early Communication Skills. North Ryde, NSW: Macquarie University.

Bodrova E, Leong DJ (1996) Tools of the Mind: The Vygotskian Approach to Early Childhood Education. Englewood Cliffs, NJ: Merrill.

Boehm AE (1986) Boehm Test of Basic Concepts – Preschool. San Antonio, Tex: Harcourt Brace Jovanovich.

Bowlby L (1982) Attachment and Loss: Vol 1 Attachment, 2nd edn. London: Hogarth.

Brennan M, Colville M, Lawson L (1984) Words in Hand – A Structural Analysis of the Signs of British Sign Language, 2nd ed. Edinburgh: Edinburgh BSL Research Project.

Bricker D (1992) The changing nature of communication and language intervention. In: Warren SF, Reichle J (eds), Causes and Effects in Communication and Language Intervention. Baltimore, Md: Brookes, pp. 361–375.

Brown AI, Metz KE, Campione JC (1996) Social interaction and individual understanding in a community of learners: the influence of Piaget and Vygostky. In: Tryphon A, Voneche J (eds), Piaget-Vygotsky: The Social Genesis of Thought. London: Psychology Press, pp. 145–170.

Brown R (1973) A First Language: The Early Stages. Cambridge, Mass: Harvard University Press.

Bruner JS (1975) From communication to language – a psychological perspective. Cognition 3, 255–287.

Bruner JS (1983) Child's Talk: Learning to Use Language. New York: Norton.

Bruner J (1999) The intentionality of referring. In: Zelazo PD, Astington JW, Olsen DR (eds), Developing Theories of Intention: Social Understanding and Self-control. Mahwah, NJ: Erlbaum, pp. 329–339.

Bruner JS, Sherwood V (1976) Peekaboo and the learning of rule structures. In: Bruner JS, Jolly A, Sylva K (eds), Play: its Role in Development and Evolution. Harmondsworth: Penguin, pp. 277–285.

Buckley S (2001) Speech and Language Development for Individuals with Down Syndrome – An Overview: Down Syndrome Issues and Information. Portsmouth: The Down Syndrome Educational Trust.

Buckley S, Bird G (2001) Speech and Language Development for Infants with Down Syndrome (0–5 years): Down Syndrome Issues and Information. Portsmouth: The Down Syndrome Educational Trust.

Bushnell IWR, Sai F, Mullin JT (1989) Neonatal recognition of the mother's face. British Journal of Developmental Psychology 7, 3–15.

Butterfield N (1994) Play as an assessment and intervention strategy for children with language and intellectual disabilities. In: Linfoot K (ed.), Communication Strategies for People with Developmental Disabilities: Issues from Theory and Practice. Sydney: MacLennan and Petty, pp. 12–44.

Chazan M, Laing A, Jackson S (1971) Just Before School: Schools Council Research and Development Project in Compensatory Education. Oxford: Blackwell.

Cherkes-Julkowski M, Gertner N (1989) Spontaneous Cognitive Processes in Handicapped Children. New York: Springer-Verlag.

Chiocca E (1998) Language development in bilingual children. Paediatric Nursing 24, 43–49.

Chomsky N (1965) Aspects of the Theory of Syntax. Cambridge, Mass: MIT Press.

Chomsky N (1986) Knowledge of Language: Its Nature, Origin and Use. New York: Praeger.

Cichetti D, Ganiban J (1990) The organization and coherence of developmental processes in the infants and children with Down syndrome. In: Hodapp RM, Burack JA, Zigler E (eds), Issues in the Developmental Approach to Mental Retardation. New York: Cambridge University Press, pp. 169–225.

Cirrin F, Rowland C (1985) Communicative assessment of nonverbal youths with severe profound mental retardation. Mental Retardation 2, 52–62.

Clark C, Davies C, Woodcock R (1974) Standard Rebus Glossary. Pine Circles, Minn: American Guidance Service.

Clarke P (1999) Investigating second language acquisition in preschool: a longitudinal study of four Vietnamese speaking children's acquisition of language in a bilingual preschool. International Journal of Early Years Education 71, 17–24.

Coggins TE, Carpenter R (1978) Categories for coding pre-speech intentional communication. Unpublished manuscript. Seattle: University of Washington.

COMPIC (1989) COMPIC: Computer Pictographs for Communication, 2nd edn. North Baldwyn, Vic: COMPIC Development Association.

Conti-Ramsden G (1994) Language interaction with atypical language learners. In: Gallaway C, Richards BJ (eds), Input and Interaction in Language Acquisition. Cambridge: Cambridge University Press, pp. 183–196.

Cooney A, Knox G (1980) Sign it and say it: a manual of New South Wales (Australian) signs for use with the Revised Makaton Vocabulary. Stockton: Stockton Hospital Welfare Association.

Cooper RP, Aslin RN (1990) Preference for infant-directed speech in the first month after birth. Child Development 61, 1584–1595.

Cromer RF (1991) Language and Thought in Normal and Handicapped Children. Oxford: Blackwell.

Cupples L (2001) The development of phonological awareness and its relationship to literacy advances. Speech-Language Pathology 3, 159–162.

Curtiss S (1977) Genie: A Psycholinguistic Study of a Modern-Day 'Wild Child'. New York: Academic Press.

Deuchar M, Quay S (2000) Bilingual Acquisition: Theoretical Implications of a Case Study. Oxford: Oxford University Press.

Dicarlo C, Banajee M (2000) Using voice output devices to increase initiations of young children with disabilities. Journal of Early Intervention 23, 191–199.

Dice K (1994) Selection of initial vocabularies for use in manual sign language programs. In: Linfoot K (ed.), Communication Strategies for People with Developmental Disabilities: Issues from Theory and Practice. Artamon: MacLennan and Petty, pp. 85–123.

Dore J (1975) Holophrases, speech acts and language universals. Journal of Child Language 2, 21–40.

Dore J (1978) Conditions for the acquisition of speech acts. In: Markova I (ed.), The Social Context of Language. Chichester: Wiley, pp. 87–111.

Duncan DM (ed.) (1989) Working with Bilingual Language Disability: Therapy in Practice. London: Chapman & Hall.

Dunn J (1999) Making sense of the social world: Mind reading, emotion, and relationships. In: Zelazo PD, Astington JW, Olson DR (eds), Developing Theories of Intention. Mahwah, NJ: Erlbaum, pp. 229–242.

Dunst CJ, Trivette CM, Deal AG (1988) Enabling and Empowering Families: Principles and Guidelines for Practice. Cambridge, MA: Brookline.

Eisenberg RB (1976) Auditory Competence in Early Life: The roots of communicative behavior. Baltimore, MD: University Park Press.

Elkind D (1990) Academic pressures – too much too soon: The demise of play. In: Klugman E, Smilansky S (eds), Children's Play and Learning: Perspectives and policy implications. New York: Teachers College Press, pp. 3–17.

Ellsworth CP, Muir DW, Hains SMJ (1993) Social competence and person-object differentiation: an analysis of the still-face effect. Developmental Psychology 29, 63–73.

Erting C, Volterra V (1990) Conclusion. In: Erting C, Volterra V (eds), From Gesture to Language in Hearing and Deaf Children. New York: Springer-Verlag, pp. 299–303.

Ferguson C (1978) Learning to pronounce: The earliest stages of phonological development in the child. In: Minifie F, Lloyd L (eds.). Communicative and Cognitive abilities – Early Behavioural Assessment. Baltimore: University Park Press, pp. 273–77.

Fernald A, Mazzie C (1991) Prosody and focus in adult speech to infants and adults. Developmental Psychology 27, 209–221.

Ferrell K (1998) Project PRISM: A longitudinal study of developmental patterns of children who are visually impaired: Final Report (CFDA 84.0203C). Greeley: University of Northern Colorado.

Fey ME, Catts HW, Larrivee LS (1995) Preparing preschoolers for the academic and social challenges of school. In: Fey ME, Windsor J, Warren SE (eds), Language Intervention: Preschool Through the Elementary Years. Baltimore, Md: Brookes, pp. 3–37.

Fletcher P, MacWhinney B (eds), (1995) The Handbook of Child Language. Oxford: Blackwell.

Fraiberg S, Smith M, Adelson E (1969) An educational program for blind infants. Journal of Special Education 3, 121–139.

Froom J, Culpepper L (1991) Otitis media in day-care children: a report from the International Primary Care network. Journal of Family Practice 32, 289–294.

Gallaway C, Richards BJ (eds) (1994) Input and Interaction in Language Acquisition. Cambridge: Cambridge University Press.

Garcia EE, DeHaven ED (1974) Use of operant techniques in the establishment and generalisation of language: a review and analysis. American Journal of Mental Deficiency 79, 169–178.

Gibbs B, Springer A (1995) Early Use of Total Communication: An Introductory Guide for Parents. Baltimore, Md: Brookes.

Goldbart J (1988) Re-examining the development of early communication. In: Coupe J, Goldbart J (eds), Communication Before Speech: Normal Development and Impaired Communication. New York: Croom Helm, pp. 19–30.

Goldin-Meadow S, Morford M (1990) Gesture in early child language. In: Erting C, Volterra V (eds), From Gesture to Language in Hearing and Deaf Children. New York: Springer-Verlag, pp. 249–262.

Goodman JF (1992) When Slow is Fast Enough: Educating the Delayed Preschool Child. New York: Guilford.

Gray BB, Ryan BP (1973) A Language Program for the Non-Language Child. Champaign, Ill: Research Press.

Greenfield PM, Smith JH (1976) Structure of Communication in Early Language Development. New York: Academic Press.

Haggard M (1995) Risk factors for otitis media: Where next? Keynote address, Australasian Conductive Deafness Association Inc, 2nd National Conference, Melbourne, 28–30 September.

Haith MM (1980) The Rules that Babies Look By: The Organization of Newborn Visual Activity. Hillsdale, NJ: Erlbaum.

Halliday M (1973) Explorations in the function of language. In: Lyons J (ed.), New Horizons in Linguistics. Harmondsworth: Penguin.

Halliday MAK (1975) Learning How to Mean: Explorations in the Development of Language. London: Edward Arnold.

Halliday MAK (1979) Development of texture in child language. In: Myers T (ed.), The Development of Conversation and Discourse. Edinburgh: Edinburgh University Press, pp. 72–87.

Harrison P, Kaufman A, Kaufman N, Bruininks R, Rynders J, Ilmer S, Sparrow C, Cicchetti D (1990) Early Screening Profiles. Circle Pines, Minn: American Guidance Service.

Hayden AH, Dmitriev V (1975) The multidisciplinary preschool program for Down's Syndrome children at the University of Washington's Model Preschool Center. In:. Friedlander B, Sterritt G, Kirk G (eds), Exceptional Infant (Vol. 3). Assessment and Intervention. New York: Brunner/Mazel, pp. 193–221.

Hedrick DL, Prather EM, Tobin AR (1995) Sequenced Inventory of Communication Development Revised (SICD-R), revised edn. Austin, TX: Pro-Ed.

Hill P, McCune-Nicolich L (1981) Pretend play and patterns of cognition in Down's syndrome infants. Child Development 52, 1168–75.

Hirsh-Pasek K, Golinkoff RM (1996) The Origins of Grammar: Evidence from Early Language Comprehension. Cambridge, MA: MIT Press.

Hoff E, Naigles L (2002) How children use input to acquire a lexicon. Child Development 73, 418–434.

Hollich GJ, Hirsh-Pasek K, Golinkoff RM (2000) Breaking the language barrier: an emergentist coalition model for the origins of word learning. Monographs of the Society for Research in Child Development 65(3).

Hondow M, Watchman J (eds) (1990) A Picture Dictionary of Australasian Signs for Young Children. Adelaide, SA: Education Department of South Australia.

Horstmeier DS, MacDonald JD (1978) Ready, Set, Go; Talk to Me: Individualised Programs for Use in Therapy, Home and Classroom. Columbus: Merrill.

Howe CJ (1993) Language Learning: A Special Case for Developmental Psychology? Hove: Erlbaum.

Hunt J McV (1961) Intelligence and Experience. New York: Ronald Press.

Hutt SJ, Tyler S, Hutt C, Christopherson H (1989) Play Exploration and Learning: A Natural History of the Pre-school. London: Routledge.

Ingram D (1978) Sensori-motor intelligence and language development. In: Lock A (ed.), Action, Gesture and Symbol: The Emergence of Language. London: Academic Press, pp. 261–290.

Ingram D (1989) First Language Acquisition: Method, Description and Explanation. Cambridge: Cambridge University Press.

Iverson JM, Thal DJ (1998) Communicative transitions: There's more to the hand than meets the eye. In: Wetherby AM, Warren SF, Reichle J (eds), Transitions in Prelinguistic Communication, Vol. 7. Baltimore, Md: Brookes, pp. 59–86.

Jaffe J, Beebe B, Feldstein S, Crown CL, Jasnow MD (2001) Rhythms of dialogue in infancy. Monographs of the Society for Research in Child Development 66(2).

Jeanes RC, Reynolds B, Coleman BC (eds) (1993) Dictionary of Australasian Signs. Melbourne, Vic: Victorian School for Deaf Children.

Johnson TA (1989) Auslan Dictionary: A Dictionary of the Sign Language of the Australian Deaf Community. Petersham, NSW: Deafness Resources Australia.

Johnson T, King D, Sloan N (1993) The Boardmaker (international) with the Picture Communication Symbols, Books I, II and III. Solana Beach, Calif: Mayer-Johnson.

Jones PR, Cregan A (1986) Sign and Symbol Communication for Mentally Handicapped People. London: Croom Helm.

Kaiser AP (1993) Parent-implemented language intervention: an environmental system perspective. In: Kaiser AP, Gray DB (eds), Enhancing Children's Communication: Research Foundations for Intervention. Communication and Language Intervention Series, Vol. 2. Baltimore, Md: Brookes, pp. 63–84.

Kaye K (1982) The Mental and Social Life of Babies: How parents create persons. Brighton: Harvestor.

Kent LR (1974) Language acquisition program for the severely retarded. Champaign, Ill: Research Press.

Kent RD, Miolo G (1995) Phonetic abilities in the first year of life. In: Fletcher P, MacWhinney B (eds), The Handbook of Child Language. Oxford: Blackwell, pp. 303–334.

Kiernan C, Reid B (1987) The Pre-verbal Communication Schedule (PVCS). Windsor: NFER/Nelson.

Kilminster MGE, Laird EM (1983) Articulation development in children aged three to nine years. Australian Journal of Human Communication Disorders 6(1), 23–30.

Knobloch H, Stevens F, Malone AF (1980) Manual of Developmental Diagnosis: The Administration and Interpretation of the Revised Gesell and Amatruda Developmental and Neurological Examination. Haggerstown, Md: Harper and Row.

Koul R, Schlosser R, Sancibrian S (2001) Effects of symbol referent and instructional variables on the acquisition of aided and unaided symbols with individuals with autism spectrum disorders. Focus on Autism and Other Developmental Disabilities 16, 162–169.

Krashen SD (1982) Principles and Practice in Second Language Acquisition. Oxford: Pergamon

Lamb ME, Campos JJ (1982) Development in Infancy: An Introduction. New York: Random House.

Legerstee M (1992) A review of the animate–inanimate distinction in infancy: implications for models of social and cognitive knowing. Early Development and Parenting 1, 59–67.

Lifter K, Bloom L (1998) Intentionality and the role of play in the transition to language. In: Wetherby AM, Warren SF, Reichle J (1998) Transitions in Prelinguistic Children, Vol. 7. Baltimore, Md: Brookes, pp. 161–195.

Linn MI, Goodman JF, Lender WL (2000) Played out? Passive behaviour by children with Down syndrome during unstructured play. Journal of Early Intervention 23, 264–278.

Lock AJ, Service V, Brito A, Chandler P (1989) The social structuring of infant cognition. In: Slater A, Bremner G (eds). Infant Development. London: Erlbaum, pp. 243–271.

Locke JL (1993) The Child's Path to Spoken Language Cambridge, Mass: Harvard University Press.

Ludemann PM (1991) Generalised discrimination of positive facial expressions by seven and ten-month-old infants. Child Development 62, 55–67.

Luze GJ, Linebarger DL, Greenwood CR, Carta JJ, Walker D, Leitschuh C, Atwater JB (2001) Developing a general outcome measure of growth in the expressive communication of infants and toddlers. School Psychology Review 30, 383–407.

Mahoney G (1988) Enhancing the developmental competence of handicapped infants. In: Marfo K (ed) Parent–Child Interaction and Developmental Disabilities: Theory, Research and Intervention. New York: Praeger, pp. 203–219.

Mahoney G, Robenalt K (1986) A comparison of conversational patterns between mothers and their Down's syndrome and normal infants. Journal of the Division of Early Childhood 10, 172–180.

Makin L (1992) Supporting children's home languages in mainstream educational programs. Australian Review of Applied Linguistics 15, 71–84.

Makin L, Campbell J, Jones Diaz C (1995) One Childhood Many Languages: Guidelines for Early Childhood Educators in Australia. Pymble, NSW: Harper Educational.

Mandler JM, Johnson NS (1977) Remembrance of things parsed: story structure and recall. Cognitive Psychology 9, 111–151.

Martinsen H, Smith L (1989) Studies of vocalisation and gesture in the transition to speech. In: von Tezchner S, Siegel LS, Smith L (eds), The Social and Cognitive Aspects of Normal and Atypical Language Development. New York: Springer-Verlag, pp. 51–68.

Masur E (1997) Maternal labelling of novel and familiar objects: Implications for children's development of lexical constraint. Journal of Child Language, 24, 427–39.

McCarthy D (1954) Language development in children. In: Carmichael L (ed) Manual of Child Psychology. New York: John Wiley, pp. 492–630.

McCollum J (1999) Parent education: What we mean and what that means. Topics in Early Childhood Education 19, 147–149.

McLean J, Snyder-McLean L (1978) A Transactional Approach to Early Language Training. Columbus, Ohio: Merrill.

McNaughton S (1975) Teaching Guidelines – Blissymbolics Communication. Fareham, Mass: Farleys.

McNeill D (1970) The Acquisition of Language: The Study of Developmental Linguistics. New York: Harper and Row.

Messer DJ (1994) The Development of Communication: From Social Interaction to Language. Chichester, West Sussex: Wiley.

Miles D (1988) British Sign Language: A beginner's guide. London: BBC Books.

Mills J (1993) Monolingual teachers assessing bilingual children. In: Mills R, Mills J (eds), Bilingualism in the Primary School. London: Routledge, pp. 59–85.

Mirenda P (2001) Autism augmentative communication and assistive technology: what do we really know? Focus on Autism and Other Developmental Disabilities 16, 141–151.

Montessori M (1967) The Absorbent Mind. New York: Holt, Rinehart and Winston.

Mowrer OH (1960) Learning Theory and Symbolic Processes. New York: John Wiley.

Muir DW, Hains SMJ (1999) Young infants' perception of adult intentionality: Adult contingency and eye direction. In: Rochat P (ed) Early Social Cognition: Understanding others in the first months of life. Mahwah, NJ: Erlbaum, pp. 155–187.

Nelson CA (1987) The recognition of facial expressions in the first year of life: mechanisms of development. Child Development. 58, 889–909.

Nelson K (1973) Structure and strategy in learning to talk. Monographs of the Society for Research in Child Development 38, 149.

Nelson K (ed.) (1986) Event Knowledge: Structure and Function in Development. Hillsdale, NJ: Erlbaum.

Nelson K (ed.) (1989) Narratives from the Crib. Cambridge, Mass: Harvard University Press.

Nelson K (1996) Language in Cognitive Development. Cambridge: Cambridge University Press.

Nelson K, Gruendel JM (1979) At morning it's lunchtime: a scriptal view of children's dialogues. Discourse Processes 2, 73–94.

Newsome M, Jusczyk PW (1995) Do infants use stress as a cue for segmenting fluent speech? In: MacLaughlin D, McEwen S (eds), 19th Boston University Conference on Language Development. Somerville, Mass: Cascadilla Press, pp. 415–426.

Nice M (1925) Length of sentences as a criterion of child's progress in speech. Journal of Educational Psychology 16, 370–9.

Nicoladis E, Secco G (2000) The role of a child's productive vocabulary in the choice of a bilingual family. First Language 20, 3–28.

Ogletree B, Harn W (2001) Augmentative and alternative communication for persons with autism: history, issues and unanswered questions. Focus on Autism and Other Developmental Disabilities 16, 138–140.

Owens RE (1996) Language Development: An Introduction, 4th edn. Needham Heights, Mass: Allyn & Bacon.

Papousek M, Papousek H, Haekel M (1987) Didactic adjustments in fathers' and mothers' speech to their three-month-old infants. Journal of Psycholinguistic Research 16, 491–516.

Paul R (2001) Language Disorders from Infancy through Adolescence: Assessment and Intervention. St Louis, Mo: Mosby.

Paul R, Fountain R (1999) Predicting outcomes of early expressive language delay. Infant Toddler Intervention 8, 123–136.

Piaget J (1962) The Language and Thought of the Child. London: Routledge and Kegan Paul.

Pieterse M (1988) The Down syndrome program at Macquarie University: a model early intervention program. In: Pieterse M, Bochner S, Bettison S (eds), Early Intervention for Children with Disabilities: The Australian Experience. Sydney, NSW: Macquarie University, pp. 81–96.

Pond R, Steiner V, Zimmerman IL (1992) Preschool Language Scale 3. San Antonio, Tex: Harcourt Brace Jovanovich.

Rahmani M (1987) Consonance. Canberra, ACT: National Library of Australia.

Ramsey P (1987) Teaching and Learning in a Diverse World. New York: Teachers College Press.

Rasore-Quantino A (1999) The present state of medical knowledge in Down syndrome. In: Rondal J, Perera J, Nadel L (eds), Down Syndrome: A Review of Current Knowledge. London: Whurr, pp. 153–162.

Ratner N, Bruner JS (1978) Games social exchange and the acquisition of language. Journal of Child Language 5, 391–401.

Reichle J, Halle J, Johnson S (1993) Developing an initial communicative repertoire: Applications and issues for persons with disabilities. In: Kaise AP, Gray DB (eds), Enhancing Children's Communication: Research Foundations for Communication, Vol. 2. Baltimore, Md: Brookes, pp. 105–136.

Reznick JS (1999) Influences on maternal attribution of infant intentionality. In: Zelazo PD, Astington JW, Olsen DR (eds), Developing Theories of Intention. Mahwah, NJ: Erlbaum, pp. 243–267.

Richards BJ, Gallaway C (1994) Conclusions and directions. In: Gallaway C, Richards B (eds), Input and Interaction in Language Acquisition. Cambridge: Cambridge University Press, pp. 253–269.

Roseberry-McKibbin C (1994) Assessment and intervention for children with limited English proficiency and language disorders. American Journal of Speech and Language Pathology 77, 77–88.

Rutter M, Rutter M (1992) Developing Minds: Challenge and Continuity across the Life Span. Harmondsworth: Penguin.

Ryan A (1996) Sign to me – speak to me: facilitating social and emotional development through the use of sign. Paper presented to the Australian Early Intervention Association (NSW Chapter) Conference: Sydney.

Salinger TS (1988) Language Arts and Literacy for Young Children. Columbus, Ohio: Merrill.

Sameroff AJ, Chandler MJ (1975) Reproductive risk and the continuum of care-taking casualty. In: Horowitz FD, Hetherington M, Seigel G (eds), Review of Child Development Research, Vol. 4. Chicago: University of Chicago Press, pp. 187–244.

Santos de Barons M, Barona A (1991) The assessment of culturally and linguistically different preschoolers. Early Childhood Research Quarterly 6, 363–377.

Sapp W (2001) Maternal perceptions of preverbal communication in children with visual impairments. Re:view 33, 133–146.

Schaeffer B (1980) Spontaneous language through signed speech. In: Schiefelbusch RL (ed), Nonspeech Language and Communication: Analysis and Intervention, pp 421–446. Baltimore: University Park Press.

Schaffer HR (1989) Language development in context. In: von Tetzchner S, Siegel LS, Smith L (eds), The Social and Cognitive Aspects of Normal and Atypical Language Development. New York: Springer-Verlag, pp. 1–22.

Searle JR (1969) Speech Acts: An Essay in the Philosophy of Language. London: Cambridge University Press.

Shank RC, Abelson RP (1977) Scripts, Plans, Goals and Understanding: An Enquiry into Human Knowledge Structures. Hillsdale, NJ: Erlbaum.

Shatz M (1987) Bootstrapping operations in child language. In: Nelson K, Van Kleeck A (eds), Children's Language, Vol. 6. Hillsdale NJ: Erlbaum, pp. 1–22.

Shriberg LD, Kwiatkowski J (1986) Natural Process Analysis: A Procedure for Phonological Analysis of Continuous Speech Samples. New York: Macmillan.

Silman S, Silverman CA (1991) Auditory Diagnosis: Principles and Applications. San Diego: Academic Press.

Simion F, Butterworth G (1998) The Development of Sensory Motor and Cognitive Capacities in Early Infancy: From Perception to Cognition. Hove, East Sussex: Psychology Press.

Skinner BF (1957) Verbal Behaviour. New York: Appleton-Century-Crofts.

Slater A (1989) Visual memory and perception in early infancy. In: Slater A, Bremner G (eds), Infant Development. London: Erlbaum, pp. 43–71.

Slater A (2000) Visual perception in the young infant: early organisation and rapid learning. In: Muir D, Slater A (eds), Infant Development: The Essential Readings. Oxford: Blackwell, pp. 95–116.

Slobin DI (1985) The Crosslinguistic Study of Language Development, Vol. 1, The Data. Hillsdale, NJ: Erlbaum.

Snow C (1994) Beginning from baby talk: Twenty years of research on input and interaction. In: Gallaway C, Richards B (eds), Input and Interaction in Language Acquisition. Cambridge: Cambridge University Press, pp. 3–12.

Snow CE (1995) Issues in the study of input: Finetuning universality individual and developmental differences and necessary causes. In: Fletcher P, MacWhinney B (eds), The Handbook of Child Language. Oxford: Blackwell, pp. 180–193.

Snyder LK, Lovitt JC, Smith JO (1975) Language training for the severely retarded: Five years of behaviour analysis research. Exceptional Children 42, 7–15.

Stern DN, Spieker S, MacKain K (1982) Intonation contours as signals in maternal speech to prelinguistic infants. Developmental Psychology 18, 727–735.

Stern W (1924) Psychology of Early Childhood up to the Sixth Year of Age. New York: Holt.

Sternberg M (1994) American Sign Language (rev. ed.). New York: Harper & Row.

Stiebel D (1999) Promoting augmentative communication during daily routines: a parent problem-solving intervention. Journal of Positive Behavior Interventions 1, 159–169.

Stoel-Gammon C (1997) Phonological development in Down syndrome. Retardation and Developmental Disability Research Reviews 3, 300–306.

Stremel K, Waryas C (1974) A behavioural-psycholinguistic approach to language training. In: McReynolds L (ed.), Developing Systematic Procedures for Training Children's Language. ASHA Monographs, No. 18. Danville, Ill: Interstate Press.

Sylva K, Bruner J, Genova P (1976) The role of play in the problem-solving of children 3–5 years old. In: Bruner J, Jolly A, Sylva K (eds), Play: Its Role in Development and Evolution. Harmondsworth: Penguin, pp. 244–257.

Sylva K, Roy C, Painter M (1980) Childwatching in Playgroup and Nursery School. London: Grant McIntyre.

Tannock R (1988) Mother's directiveness in their interactions with their children with and without Down's syndrome. American Journal of Mental Retardation 93, 154–165.

Thompson RA (1998) Early sociopersonality development. In: Eisenberg N (ed) Handbook of Child Psychology, Vol. 3. Social, Emotional and Personality Development, 5th edn. New York: Wiley, pp. 25–104.

Tizard B, Hodges J (1978) The effects of early institutional rearing on the development of eight year old children. Journal of Child Psychology and Psychiatry 10, 99–118.

Tomasello M (1992) First Verbs: Case Study of Early Grammatical Development. Cambridge: Cambridge University Press.

Tomasello M (2001) Perceiving intentions and learning words in the second year of life. In: Bowerman M, Levinson S (eds), Language Acquisition and Conceptual Development. Cambridge: Cambridge University Press, pp. 132–158.

Tomasello M, Mannle S, Kruger AC (1986) Linguistic environment of 1- to 2-year-old twins. Developmental Psychology 22, 169–176.

Toppelberg C, Snow C, Tager-Flusberg H (1999) Several developmental disorders and bilingualism. Journal of the American Academy of Child and Adolescent Psychiatry 10, 197–200.

Trehub SE, Thorpe LA (1989) Infants' perception of rhythm: categorization of auditory sequences by temporal structures. Canadian Journal of Psychology 43, 217–229.

Trevarthen C (1979) Communication and co-operation in early infancy: A description of early intersubjectivity. In: Bullowa M (ed.), Before Speech: The Beginning of Interpersonal Communication. Cambridge: Cambridge University Press, pp. 321–347.

Turnbull A, Blue-Banning M, Turbiville V, Park J (1999) From parent education to partnership education: A call for a transformed focus. Topics in Early Childhood Education 19, 164–174.

Uzgiris I, Hunt J McV (1989) Assessment in Infancy: Ordinal Scales of Infant Psychological Development. Urbana, Ill: University of Illinois Press.

von Tetzchner S, Martinsen H (2000) Introduction to Augmentative and Alternative Communication, 2nd edn. London: Whurr.

Vygotsky L.S (1978). Mind in Society: The Development of Higher Mental Processes. Cambridge, Mass: Harvard University Press (eds Cole M. John-Steiner V, Scribner S, Souberman E; originally published 1930).

Vygotsky LS (1986) Thought and Language. Cambridge, Mass: MIT Press. (trans. Kozulin A, from the original work published posthumously in 1934).

Wadsworth BJ (1996) Piaget's Theory of Cognitive and Affective Development: Foundations of Constructivism, 5th edn. White Plains, NY: Longman.

Walton GE, Bower NJ, Bower TGR (1992) Recognition of familiar faces by newborns. Infant Behaviour and Development 15, 265–269.

Ward J (1997) Foreword. In: Bochner S, Price P, Jones J, Child Language Development: Learning to Talk. London: Whurr.

Warren SF, Yoder PJ (1998) Facilitating the transition from preintentional to intentional communication. In: Wetherby A, Warren S, Reichle J (eds), Transitions in Prelinguistic Communication, Vol. 7. Baltimore, Md: Brookes, pp. 365–84.

Wells G (1985) Language Development in the Preschool Years. Cambridge: Cambridge University Press.

Werner H, Kaplan B (1963) Symbol Formation: An Organismic-Developmental Approach to Language and the Expression of Thought. New York: Wiley.

Wetherby AM, Prizant BM (1989) The expression of communicative intent: assessment guidelines. Seminars in Speech and Language 10, 77–91.

Wetherby AM, Warren SF, Reichle J (1998) Transitions in Prelinguistic Communication, Vol. 7. Baltimore, MD: Brookes.

Wilcox MJ, Shannon MS (1998) Facilitating the transition from prelinguistic to linguistic communication. In: Wetherby A, Warren S, Reichle J (eds), Transitions in Prelinguistic Communication, Vol. 7. Baltimore, Md: Brookes, pp. 385–416.

Winitz H (1969) Articulatory Acquisition and Behaviour. New York: Appleton-Century-Crofts.

Woollett A (1986) The influence of older siblings in the language environment of young children. British Journal of Developmental Psychology 4, 235–245.

Yoder PJ, Warren SF (2001) Relative treatment effects of two prelinguistic communication interventions on language development in toddlers with developmental delays vary by maternal characteristics. Journal of Speech, Language and Hearing Research 44, 224–237.

Yoder PJ, Warren SF, McCathren R, Leew SV (1998) Does adult responsivity to child behaviour facilitate communication development? In: Wetherly AM, Warren SF, Reichle J (eds), Transitions in Prelinguistic Communication, Vol. 7. Baltimore, Md: Brookes, pp. 39–56.

Zelazo PD, Astington JW, Olsen DR (eds) (1999) Developing Theories of Intention: Social Understanding and Self control. Mahwah, NJ: Erlbaum.

Appendix A
Language sampling

A language sample gives useful information on how a child is communicating and on the appropriateness of your language. This information is particularly useful for children who are just starting to talk.

Taking a language sample

- Set up a situation where you can play with the child using toys or books that you know the child enjoys. Dolls and a tea-set, or a barn with animals, have been shown to be particularly effective for encouraging children to communicate (Luze et al., 2001).
- Once you begin to play with the materials, try to say nothing for the first few minutes. Play alongside the child at first, in parallel play mode, following the child's lead rather than directing the activity. This will give the child an opportunity to demonstrate his or her communication skills without prompting from you. After a few minutes, you can begin to play more interactively. Follow the child's lead and talk with the child about what you are doing.
- Record your play together for 5–10 minutes using a video- or audio-tape recorder.

Transcribing a language sample

The following guidelines should be helpful:

- Listen to the tape or watch the video recording and write down every communicative act produced by the child. You can also record your own communication. An act can take the form of eye movements (attention to you or to an object or action), gestures, signs or other actions, sounds or utterances made by either you or the child. An utterance need not be a complete sentence. If there is a longish pause, write the next words said as a new utterance.

- Use a new line for each communicative act or utterance.
- Write the child's and adult's acts or utterances in different colours.
- Note whether any utterances take the form of, or are accompanied by, a meaningful gesture (G) or sign (S).

Be sure to write down exactly what is said or observed, not what you expect to hear or see. Sometimes the child's speech may not be clear. Write exactly what the child says and put the correct form of the word afterwards in brackets. If the child makes only sounds, try to record these. Table A.1 shows two examples recorded while a parent and child were reading a book together.

Table A.1 Two recorded language samples

Example 1	
Adult:	(pointing) 'that's a car'
Child:	'car'
Adult:	'push car'
Child:	(touching picture) 'br'mm br'mm' (+G)
Example 2	
Child:	'drink' (+S)
Adult:	'drink milk'
Child:	(drinking sound)
Adult:	'all gone?'
Child:	'all gone' (+G)

Analyse the language sample to gain information about your own behaviour and language and that of the child. This can include calculation of the ratio of adult–child utterances and the mean length of utterance (MLU) of the child.

Ratio of adult–child utterances

Count the number of utterances spoken by you and the number spoken by the child. If the ratio is more than 2 : 1 (if there were twice as many utterances by the adult when compared with those of the child), then you are probably talking too much and not giving the child enough opportunity to speak. For example:

- total child utterances: 51
- total adult utterances: 107 ratio 2 : 1 (acceptable)
- total adult utterances: 150 ratio 3 : 1 (too many words)

Calculating the mean length of utterance

To calculate an MLU, count the number of words spoken and divide this by the number of utterances (sentences or part-sentences) spoken. Do not include signs or gestures here. Calculate the MLU separately for adult and child. If your own MLU is more than a couple of words longer than that of the child, take care to keep your utterances short and simple. For example:

- child MLU: 1.3
- adult MLU: 3.1 (acceptable)
- adult MLU: 5.6 (too many words)

If the child is using a number of signs, sounds and gestures, you may wish to keep a record of the number used during the language sample. You will expect this number to decrease as more intelligible words are uttered. Keep a record of:

- total number of signs
- total number of sounds
- total number of gestures.

If the child uses a mixture of intelligible and unintelligible words, it may be useful also to calculate an MLU for intelligible utterances. This is done by dividing the total number of intelligible words by the total number of utterances, as in the following example:

- total number of intelligible words:		39

- total number of utterances:			32

- MLU (intelligible):				1.2

Appendix B
Summary assessment sheets

Level 1: Preliminary skills

Looking together

Child's name _____ *Date* _____

- Criterion: child is involved in joint attention with adult for at least five seconds.
- Procedure: engage child in activity that should attract his or her attention. Encourage the child to look.
- Materials: pop-up toy; toy car in bag; picture book or pull-along toy; bell in box; glove puppet; simple pictures.
- Scoring child's response: yes = 1 no = 0

Looking together tasks	Child's response	Comment	Alternative tasks
Pop-up toy			Pull-along toy
Toy in bag			Bell in box
Finger play			Puppet talks to child
Picture book			Simple pictures
Total			

- Achieved: 3 out of 4 tasks
- Emerging: If only 1 or 2 tasks are achieved, give more practice.
- Not yet ready: If no tasks are achieved, you should encourage eye contact and tracking or following a moving object.

Turn-taking and imitation

Child's name _____ *Date* _____

- Criterion: child takes a turn or imitates an action or sound in an activity with an adult.
- Procedure: adult introduces game and invites child to participate, saying 'do this' or 'your turn', 'my turn'.
- Materials: cloth, car, five blocks or toy and cloth, small bean bag, peg board.
- Scoring child's response: Yes = 1   No = 0
- Note sound/word approximations used in conjunction with actions

Tasks	Child's response	Did child need practice?	Alternative tasks
Turn-taking Push car			Knock over block tower
Build block tower			Throw bean bag or take pegs off board
Imitation Hide face, then uncover			Hide toy under cloth, look for it
Clap hands			Hit drum
Hit table			Tap head
Rub tummy			Wave fingers
Drop toy			Stamp foot
Total			

- Achieved: 3 out of 4 tasks, including at least 2 imitation tasks
- Emerging: If 1 or 2 of the tasks are achieved, give more practice
- Not yet ready: If no tasks are achieved, give more practice in Looking together activities

Appropriate play

Child's name _____ *Date* _____

- Criterion: child plays appropriately with objects, either functionally or imaginatively.
- Procedure: present items to child. If necessary, say 'Look, you play' or 'What can you do with this/these?'
- Materials: car, hairbrush, teapot and cup, book or animal, bowl and spoon, paper and crayon.
- Scoring child's response: Yes = 1 No = 0

Appropriate play tasks	Child's response	Did child need practice?	Alternative tasks
Toy car			Toy animal
Hairbrush			Cup
Teapot and cup			Bowl and spoon
Book			Paper and crayon
Total			

- Achieved: 3 out of 4 tasks
- Emerging: If 1 or 2 tasks are achieved with or without practice, give more practice.
- Not yet ready: If no tasks are achieved, give more practice in looking together and/or turn-taking and imitation skills.

Level 2: Preverbal skills

Performative sounds

Child's name _____ *Date* _____

- Criterion: child produces performative sounds during play.
- Procedure: introduce a game, make an appropriate sound during the game and encourage the child to imitate you.
- Materials: model cars or aeroplanes, model animals or doll and tea set, musical instruments.

Tasks	Child's response	Did child need prompt to achieve?	Alternative tasks
Peek-a-boo			Ring-a-Rosie
Model cars, animals			Tea-set and doll
Model animals			Musical instruments
Total			

- Achieved: If the child achieved 2 out of 3 tasks, go to the next level in the programme (Level 3).
- Emerging: If only 1 task was achieved, give more practice.
- Not yet ready: If no tasks were achieved, go back to Imitation and Turn-taking skills in the previous level in the programme (Level 1).

Communicative intentions using actions, gestures and sounds

Child's name _____ *Date* _____

- Criterion: child uses actions, gestures, signs or sounds to communicate intentionally.

Note: This skill can be assessed while assessing other preliminary and pre-verbal skills.

- Procedure: While playing with the child:
  1. Introduce a favourite or interesting new toy. Does the child attempt to draw your attention to it?
  2. Gently remove a toy the child is playing with so it is still in sight but out of the child's reach. Does the child protest and/or try to regain the toy?
  3. While the child is playing with a favourite toy, attempt to replace it with a less favoured object. Does the child attempt to reject the new object?
  4. Activate a pop up or musical toy in front of the child. Keep your hand near the toy but do not maintain attention to the child or toy. When the toy stops do nothing. Does the child attempt to gain your attention in any way?
- Mode: Action (A) Gesture (G) Sound (So)
- Achieved: 3 out of 4 intentions observed.
- Emerging: if only 1 or 2 intentions are observed, encourage child to express further intentions in appropriate contexts
- Not yet ready: if no intentions observed, encourage child to express intentions in appropriate contexts

Communicative intention	No. of instances observed	Example	Mode
To indicate			
To obtain desired objects or services			
To regulate actions: • protest • reject • request attention			
To initiate, maintain or terminate social interaction			

Level 3: First words

Child's name _____ *Date* _____

- Criterion: child produces single words during play.
- Procedure: introduce a game, model appropriate words and encourage child to talk.
- Materials: large cloth or paper bag, small familiar toys as listed or simple picture book.
- Scoring child's response: yes = 1 no = 0

Tasks	Child's response	Did child need prompt to achieve?	Alternative tasks
Spontaneous speech (child must label 3 to achieve this item)			
Ball			Shoe
Car			Doll
Bat			Hat
(Fall) Down			Key
Imitated speech (child must label 3 to achieve this item)			
Bell			Train or pom pom
Bird			Duck or mop
More			Dog or mat
Mum			Pig or owl
Total			

- Achieved: If child achieved 3 out of 4 tasks in both spontaneous and imitated speech, go to the next chapter on early sentences (Level 4).
- Emerging: If 1 or 2 tasks achieved in either mode, give more practice.
- Not yet ready: If no tasks were achieved in either mode, go back to the previous level in the programme (Level 2).

Note: Developmentally appropriate single syllable words may be substituted for both spontaneous and imitated speech for children whose first language is not English. For ideas on choosing words starting with appropriate consonant sounds, see Chapter 11 on phonological development.

Level 4: Early sentences

Child's name _____ *Date* _____

Early sentence rules	No. of instances observed	Percentage use
Agent + action		
Action + object		
Agent + object		
Modifier (possession) + object		
Modifier (recurrence) + object		
Modifier (attribution) + object		
Agent/object + location		
Action + location		
Negation + any word		
Introducer + any word		
Total		

Level 5: Communicative intentions using words

Child's name _____ *Date* _____

Communication mode: word = W, sign = Si, phrase or sentence = P

Communicative intention	No. of instances observed	Examples	Mode
To indicate			
To obtain desired objects or services			
To regulate actions: • protest • reject • request attention			
To initiate, maintain or terminate social interaction			
To obtain information by asking questions			
To discover new words			
To give information			
To answer questions			

• Note: Children who are using words or signs but who are not yet using them to communicate intentions should be encouraged to use appropriate words or signs in context.

English morphemes

Child's name _____ *Date* _____

Morpheme	Specific form	No. of instances observed	Percentage use
Present progressive	-ing		
Preposition	In		
Preposition	On		
Plural (regular)	-s, -es, etc.		
Past (irregular)	Came, ran, etc.		
possessive	-'s		
Uncontractible copula	is, am, are, as in 'is it blue?'		
Articles	a, the		
Past regular	-d, -ed, -/t/		
Third person regular	-s, -/z/, etc., as in 'she runs'		
Third person irregular	Does, has, as in 'They do' vs 'She does'		
Uncontractible auxiliary	is, am, are, as in 'is she running?'		
Contractible copula	-'s, -'m, -'re, as in 'it's blue'		
Contractible auxiliary	-'s, -n, -e, as in 'they're running'		
Total			

MLU	Morphemes acquired
2.0 to 2.5	-ing, in, on
2.5 to 3.0	past irregular, possessive 's, uncontracted copula
3.0 to 3.7	articles, regular past, 3rd person regular
3.7 to 4.5	3rd person irregular, uncontracted auxiliary, contracted copula, contracted progressive auxiliary

Appendix C
Observation record forms

Analysis of gestures

Child's name _____ *Date* _____

Form (describe physical action or gesture)	Meaning or intention	Date first used

Single words

Child's name _____ *Date* _____

Spontaneous = S; Imitation = I

Word	S/I	Date first used	To whom?	What was going on?	What was the child trying to say?	Was the word used again frequently?

Phrases of two, three or more words

Child's name _____ Date _____

Phrase	Date first used	To whom?	What was going on?	What was the child trying to say?	Was the phrase used again frequently?

Sounds, gestures, words or phrases

Child's name _____ *Date* _____

Communication mode: Sound = S; Gesture = G; Word = W; Phrase = P

Word Mode: S/G/W/P	Date first used	To whom?	What was going on?	What was the child trying to say?	Was this used again often?

Communication Planner – Record

Child's name _____ *Date* _____

Target	Strategies	Arrival/ Departure	Meal/snack Times	Routines	Group times	Structured Planned Activities	Unstructured Free Play Activities

Use this form to identify and record progress on individual language targets for children in a group situation

Appendix D
List of first words

Child's name _____ *Date* _____

Speech mode: spontaneous = S, imitation = I

People	S/I	Objects	S/I	Location	S/I	Action	S/I	Modifiers	S/I	Other	S/I
Family		Banana		Up		Kiss		More		Bye-bye	
Mummy		Apple		Down		Sleep		My		Hi	
Daddy		Orange		There		Want		Mine		Hello	
Baby		Bickie		Here		Wash		Your		No	
		Lolly		In		Eat		Big		Please	
		Cup		Out		Drink		Little		Thanks	
		Spoon		On		Sit		Hot		Ta	
(child's		Nose		Off		Down		Wet		Ni-night	
name)		Eye				Fall		Yuk		Goodnight	
		Comb				Comb		That			
Teachers		Shoe				Brush		This		Other	
		Sock				Gone		A		words:	
		Chair				All-gone				That	
Carers		Bath				Go				This	
		Bed				Stop					
		Door				Throw					
		Key				Up					
		Ball				In					

Child's name _____ *Date* _____

Speech mode: spontaneous = S, imitation = I

People	S/I	Objects	S/I	Location	S/I	Action	S/I	Modifiers	S/I	Other	S/I
Pets		Teddy				Do					
		Dolly				Open					
		Dog				Come					
		Book				Look					
Favourite		Bike				Point					
toys		Bus				Jump					
		Car				Help					
		Clock									
Pronouns:		Light									
Me		TV									
I		Clock									
You		Tree									
Mine											

Appendix E
Articulation development and Australian norms

Age (years;months) at which 75% accuracy is expected													
3	h	ŋ	p	m	w	b	n	d	t	j	k	g	ʒ
3;6	f												
4	l	ʃ	tʃ										
4;6	s	z	dʒ										
5	r												
6	v												
8	ð												
8;6	θ												

Phonetic symbol	Key words Initial	Medial	Final
h	Hat	Behind	
ŋ		Singer	Wing
p	Pie	Happy	Top
m	Me	Coming	Some
w	Wet	Hour	
b	Be	Cubby	Rub
n	No	Funny	When
d	Do	Muddy	Said
t	Tie	Letter	Cat
j	You	Beyond	
k	Key	Pocket	Like
g	Go	Bigger	Leg
ʒ		Measure	
f	Fun	Coffee	Laugh
l	Leg	Follow	Ball
ʃ	She	Pushing	Wash
tʃ	Chin	Kitchen	Watch
s	See	Pussy	Mess
z	Zoo	Easy	Hose
dʒ	Jump	Magic	Edge
r	Run	Borrow	
v	Vest	Ever	Stove
ð	This	Other	Smooth
θ	Thumb	Nothing	Both

Source: Kilminister and Laird (1983).

Appendix F
Resources for use in a parent-based programme

The materials included here are resources that may be used in a parent-oriented early language programme as information sheets for the parents.

- *Developmental levels in learning to talk.* This provides a description of the levels that children pass through as they acquire language.
- *Talking with children.* This reviews some of the ways in which adults can assist children to begin to communicate more effectively. Ideas for communicating with infants and young children at the prelinguistic stage are identified and strategies are suggested to use when interacting with young children who are learning to talk
- *Encouraging play.* This is an introduction to the concept of play and to the ways in which adults can interact with their children to develop appropriate play skills and, at the same time, encourage early language.
- *The parent inventory.* this is a list of questions designed to elicit basic information about the child and his or her current language skills at home. Information is also sought about parents' main concerns and expectations for the child. Parents are also asked to complete some simple observation tasks based on the type of activities that are included at each stage of the language program. The Inventory was developed from the Oliver, a parent information form associated with Horstmeier and MacDonald (1978).

Developmental language levels

Learning to talk can be compared to learning to climb a ladder. Each step on the ladder represents a new set of skills. When a child is in the early levels of learning to communicate, you can watch for signs of movement from one step to the next. Here are descriptions of the steps that children have to climb when their communication skills begin to develop (earlier summarized in Table 2.1).

Pre-programme level: uncontrolled vocalizing

Initially infants' vocalizing is largely triggered by physical events. They cry because of hunger or pain. Soon they learn to vocalize for their own entertainment with squeals and gurgles when left alone in the cot. These sounds are often interpreted as meaningful by carers, but there is no evidence that the babies produce such sounds intentionally, to convey a message.

Level 1: Preliminary skills: looking together, imitation and appropriate play

As infants develop, they acquire increasingly complex sets of behaviour for exploring their environment, learning about objects and people, and playing. Initially they usually mouth most objects but they gradually learn to bang, throw or wave them. These play strategies become increasingly complex. They learn to put small objects inside larger ones, or to bang two objects together to create an interesting effect. Some of these actions are learned by accident while others are learned while interacting with familiar adults, in games that involve both attending to something of interest, as well as imitation and turn-taking.

Level 2: Preverbal skills: gestures, performatives and protowords

Gestures

When children first want to communicate, they often use gestures that may involve hands, fingers, face and the whole body. These gestures are often accompanied by a vocalization and at the same time, children will also look at your eyes. Early gestures are used to show you something interesting such as a bird or the moon, or to represent an event such as waving goodbye or stretching out the arms and running and 'dipping' to represent an aeroplane.

Performatives

Early play routines often include a sound within a set of actions, such as 'ee-er' to accompany a pop-up toy or 'oops' when the doll falls off the table. These consistent sounds associated with actions are called performatives.

Many early sounds appear to be imitations of interesting noises heard by the child, such as 'ding ding' (telephone), 'toot toot' (bus or car), or a tongue click (bird). Other sounds reflect familiar speech patterns such as lip-smacking for preferred food, humming when tired and ready for bed, or 'oh oh' when someone falls over.

Protowords

The earliest signs of language appear when the infant begins to combine contact with objects and interactions with adults in one event. For example, the infant has watched entranced as a wind-up car turned circles for some time and has also often watched Daddy wind up a toy to activate it. The signs of early language appear when the child attempts to attract the father's attention to wind up the toy by using a consistent gesture or sound. These early consistent word-like sounds are called protowords.

Some children create their own word-like sounds for particular experiences. These are used consistently with familiar adults, who understand the meaning of the sounds. Normally such protowords are abandoned as the child learns to use more conventional word forms, as when 'car' replaces 'br'mm br'mm' or 'bottle' is used instead of a sucking noise.

Level 3: First words

Children's' first words are usually associated with experiences that have a high level of interest for them. For example, they often label things that move or change ('gone'), make a noise ('car') and are colourful ('balloon'). Words are used first to draw the attention of an adult to events of high interest ('plane', 'bird'). Later, they use words in other ways; for example, to reject an invitation ('no' to avoid a bath) or to obtain an object or help with something ('ball' to get a ball or to play with it in a game).

Most first words are labels for objects and people, though a range of other words are also acquired to represent actions ('ride'), states ('wet'), attributes ('big') and other meanings ('bye', 'more').

Level 4: Combining words: putting two words together and early sentences

Once children have about 30 or more words of various types, they begin to combine them into simple sentences. The way they sequence these words directly reflects their experiences or perception of the world. Initially they use single words to represent a variety of meanings: for example, 'drink' can mean a glass of milk or the act of drinking. Later, more explicit action words are acquired, such as 'want' and 'go'. These are eventually paired with labels to make simple sentences like 'want drink', 'go car' and 'Mummy car', or phrases like 'my car' and 'big ball'.

After children have learned to combine two words to express a variety of meanings, they begin to string more words together to produce longer sentences, such as:

'me want' + 'want drink' = 'me want drink'.
'go car' + 'Mummy car' = 'go Mummy car'

At this level children start to express more detailed information by adding words for colour, size, possession and so on, as in 'me go big red car', 'want blue ball'.

When the child has achieved these skills, it may be claimed that the basic elements of the language system have been acquired.

Level 5: Extending meaning: communicative intentions and morphology

Once children are using sentences of three or four words, they begin to use parts of the adult grammar system to indicate, for example, plurals, present and past tense, as in words such as 'cars', 'running', 'goed' (went) and 'fell'. They now add 's' to indicate possession, as in 'Daddy's car' and will contract words by saying 'She's there' or 'I'm here'.

Once children have reached this level on the language-learning ladder, they have mastered the most difficult tasks in learning to talk. Future progress will involve learning more words, more complex grammar and more sophisticated use of language skills.

Talking with children

The language that adults use when talking with young children is very important for early language learning. Parents and other regular carers have a vital role to play in this process. They direct children's attention to objects and events in the environment; help them learn to take turns in early games that involve actions and sounds; name people, objects and activities that are significant in the daily routine and praise, encourage and correct early attempts to master the language. When children are experiencing difficulties in the early stages of learning to talk, it becomes even more important that parents and regular carers use appropriate language and strategies to encourage them to talk.

Many studies have shown that the way adults talk to young children is different from the way they talk to other adults. They tend to talk more slowly, and use fewer words and simpler sentences with more repetitions. Gestures such as pointing are often used to help clarify what the adult is talking about.

Adults often take part in 'games' with children involving repeated sounds, actions and routines, extending their expectations as the children grow more competent. These and other techniques help make the child's task of learning to talk a little easier. Some suggestions about what adults can do to help children are listed below.

Gain the child's attention

It is important that we have children's attention when we are trying to tell them something. If they do not know that we are speaking to them, they may not 'turn on' to our speech. Simply calling the child's name or making sure he is looking before telling him something can be helpful.

Speak slowly and clearly

If we speak too fast, children may not be able to distinguish the individual words that let them know what we are talking about. Talking slowly and clearly lets them distinguish the words they will need to learn to say.

Avoid talking too much

The more you talk, the less opportunity the child has to say something or to take part in any conversation. When you do say something to a child, give her time to respond. Children learning to talk often need more time than we do to recognize what we have said and to work out an appropriate response. Remember, the more a child has the opportunity to talk, the more she learns about how to use language.

Use simple words

Use short simple words where possible to describe the objects and actions the child is engaged in during daily routines and other experiences such as:

'teddy', 'ball', 'cup', 'drink', 'dog', 'give', 'jump', 'run', 'sit'

It is often a good idea to leave out the little words like 'a' and 'the' in the early stages of learning when children are using only sounds or one or two words. This will help the child to focus on the main words that give meaning, for example:

'drink milk' rather than 'drink your milk'
'open door' rather than 'please open the door for me'

As your child gains confidence and puts words together into short sentences, you can add in the little words.

Take part in shared activities with the child

Children's early language learning takes place through frequent repetitions of familiar routines that involve a shared activity and turn taking with familiar adults or other children. These activities can be special play times or routine activities during the day. Examples include:

- 'Peek-a-boo' games
- saying goodnight to the family
- having a drink or snack together
- looking together at a picture book.

Comment on what the child does

Use simple sentences to comment on what the child is doing, or what you are doing together. This provides your child with the language needed to talk about things and activities that interest him. Children learn faster when they are engaged in something they have chosen. Follow the child's lead when possible rather than imposing *your* ideas, using comments like:

'Yes, wash teddy'
'Teddy sleep'
'Goodnight teddy'
'Sh-sh; sleep tight'.

Use visual prompts

Children learning to talk often find it easier to understand what we are saying to them when they can see what we are talking about. Some children need this visual support more than others. Try using objects, pictures or actions such as pointing as you speak to help the child understand what you are talking about or what you want her to do, as in:

- Point to the floor or book as you say 'Look, there's the ball'
- Show your child both fruits as you ask 'Do you want banana or pear?'
- Pat the chair to show your child where you want her to sit as you say 'sit next to me'

Extend the child's language

Extensions are statements that provide a little bit more information than was contained in the child's statement. They allow the child to hear new words that can gradually be included in utterances, as more words are used together. When responding or talking to your child, try to provide a model for expanding the next step he will be talking. For example:

- If the child says 'Teddy eat', you say 'Teddy eat toast'
- If the child says 'Teddy sleep', you say 'Teddy's sleeping'.

The expansion acknowledges what the child has already said, and extends it a little bit further, providing a model for the child's next turn, or for use in a later conversation.

A good rule to follow in deciding how long your expanded sentence should be is to use as many words as your child uses, plus one or two more.

Avoid too many questions or commands

Questions

Questions are a great way of engaging children's attention. However, if you are constantly giving instructions or asking questions, the child will be busy trying to do what you want and you will be missing opportunities for him to talk to you about the things that he likes or wants to do.

Some questions restrict the type of answer that is appropriate, such as questions that can be answered only with a 'yes' or 'no'. Try to use open questions that allow the child to express what he thinks or wants, as in:

- 'What can you see?'
- 'What happened?'
- 'Where shall we put teddy?'
- 'What's Daddy doing'

Some children find it easier to answer questions that offer a choice to start off. For example, you can ask:

- 'Do you want milk or juice?'
- 'Shall we play cars or read a book?'

As the child learns to answer these kinds of questions, you can start asking open questions, such as 'What do you want?' or 'What shall we do now?' and 'What shall we eat?' Remember to give the child time to respond.

Commands

Too many commands reduce the child's opportunity to choose a topic and to talk about what is of interest. However, there are situations where commands or directions are needed to attract the child's attention and to encourage him to join in a game or activity. This may be particularly true for slower, more passive children, or those with difficult behaviours. A balance is needed, and using an enthusiastic tone of voice will help.

Encourage the child to talk

Make sure the child knows that she is doing well, that the conversations and games shared with others are appreciated. Make the child feel worthwhile and valued. Encourage every attempt to communicate. Show your interest in what she is doing by responding to or commenting on what is happening. For example:

- 'Yes, it's a blue cup'
- 'That's right, push car. Br'mm'.

This will encourage the child to feel that her contribution is valued and of interest.

Coax the child to talk more

Sometimes children who are just learning to talk are not quite sure of the words to use in an activity and can be helped by being given part of the sentence, as in:

- 'Give the ball to . . . (Mummy)'
- 'Do you want some more . . . (juice)'

If you are not sure about the best words to use, listen and make a list of the words you hear the child use during the day. You can then use these words to encourage your child to talk more. For example, if your child uses words like 'more', or 'jump', you can show the juice and say 'You want . . . (more)', or 'Now you're going to . . . (jump)' as you hold him or her ready to jump.

Avoid correcting the child's speech

Learning to talk is a complex task. Some sounds and words are more difficult to say than others and words can come out in the wrong order. But if the focus is on the errors and the child is constantly criticized, he may become discouraged and unwilling to make future attempts. A better way of dealing with such errors is to acknowledge what the child has said and model the correct version. For example:

- If the child says 'It's big ephalent', you could say 'Yes, it's a big grey elephant'.
- If the child says 'Big sep', you could say 'Oh dear, it is a big step.'

Remember, children who are learning to talk need to hear clear models of words and to have plenty of opportunities to practise using their words in as many situations as possible. The way we talk to them is important in all their usual settings – in the home, at playgroup and daycare, and in the wider community. It is important to remember that communication involves interaction between the child and key adults, and that the way these adults talk to the child can make the child's task of learning to talk much easier. By being involved in your child's activities you will not only have more opportunities to help him or her learn to talk, you will probably find you are both enjoying yourselves.

Encouraging play

Play is an important part of each child's development. In the process of learning to play, children go through a variety of stages, from very simple exploration of objects to more complex representational or 'pretend' play where they take on a variety of roles. Examples of 'pretend' play include games such as 'mothers and fathers' or 'cops and robbers'. Through these play activities, children are able to explore and learn about the environment and their place in it. Play is used to help them adjust to new situations, such as the birth of a new baby, and to understand relationships, as in games that involve re-enacting familiar domestic situations. They also learn how to interact socially with peers, to communicate with them, resolve disagreements and develop friendships.

Over the years of their development, children need to progress through each of the stages of play. However, some children, particularly those experiencing difficulties in other aspects of development, sometimes seem to become stuck at a particular level. When this happens, you may need to encourage and help them learn more complex play skills. So it is important that you think about your role in helping children learn to play.

It has been said that play is children's work, but children can very quickly 'switch off' if we approach a play activity as if it is work. Work means effort and doing what someone else wants, whereas play should be something that you do because you want to do it. It should be flexible and, above all, it should be fun. Since many early language skills are acquired through play, you also need to ensure that you encourage play activities that will support the acquisition of these skills.

For very small children, the world must often seem large and forbidding. They need to be near their mother or someone familiar for support and security. They will follow you around as you work, often getting in your way, whining for you to notice them. If you sit down, they will come and beg for your attention. This is often a good time to stop what you are doing and play for a little while.

If you find it difficult to play, try following these suggestions:

- Begin by just sitting near the child while she is playing quietly. If you possibly can, get down on the floor, close to the child. If this feels strange to you, try sitting down with something to do that makes you feel comfortable and at ease, such as a magazine or some other simple activity.
- When your child is happily playing, look at what he is doing. The child will be happy that you are near, showing interest and approval.
- After a while, the child will approach you, perhaps to show you a toy. You can then comment on what has been happening in the game. Soon, you will be following the child's lead, playing happily together. You will both have a sense of closeness when you share an activity in this way.

- At this stage, remember to stop, watch and listen to the child while you spend time together.

Now you can begin to guide and extend the child in play. Once you and your child are comfortable sitting together and playing, you can start introducing new toys and actions, and new ways of using familiar toys. Using daily routines from home such as eating dinner, having a bath and going to bed is a good way to encourage your child to enjoy the time with you. Games that you can play include:

- taking turns to feed and bath teddy and put him to bed
- making a bridge for the cars to drive back and forth under
- throwing a ball back and forth.

These simple turn-taking routines will encourage the child to play with you and develop new play skills.

- When looking at a book, remember to talk about the pictures and point to anything of interest, rather than simply reading the words. This will encourage more communication from the child.
- Do not expect the child to follow your every idea, and give encouragement whenever she discovers new ways of doing things, without your help.
- As you play, remember to comment on what you and the child are doing. Include appropriate gestures and sounds in the game and encourage the child to imitate you or use these 'performative' sounds while playing. These are important forerunners of the words that the child will eventually start to use.

At this stage you will need a variety of things to play with so that the child can choose what is of interest. These need not be expensive. They can include:

- blocks, balls, old containers that small objects can be put into
- things to roll and shake
- cloths that can be used as blankets or to play peek-a-boo
- old plastic and cardboard containers and kitchen utensils.

Items such as these are all acceptable to children. It is a good idea to have a box or cupboard where the child can have ready access and is free to explore these toys. New objects can be added from time to time. Items that are broken or are no longer of interest can be removed. Select simple toys that are easy to manipulate and interest the child. This will avoid or lessen the inevitable frustration that comes with a toy that is too difficult or complicated. It will also enable you to build up a positive and happy relationship in which the child wants to learn from you.

Happy playing!

Parent inventory

Today's date: _____ Who is completing the report: _____
Address: _____Phone: _____

Child's name: _____Birthdate: _____
Brothers' and sisters' names: _____ _____ _____
Ages: _____ _____ _____
Mother's name: _____ Father's name: _____
Phone:_____ Phone: _____
If English is not the only language spoken in child's home, what other languages are spoken?:

_____

Is your child currently in a playgroup, preschool, nursery school or class or other early childhood
programme?   Yes ☐   No ☐   If yes,
Name of centre: _____
Address: _____
Teacher's name: _____ Phone: _____

Who plays best with the child?   _____
Who else spends a good deal of time with the child? (relatives, siblings, friends, teachers):

_____

What are your child's favourite toys? _____
What does your child enjoy doing?_____
What does your child like to eat or drink? _____

Has your child's hearing or sight been tested?   Yes ☐   No ☐
If yes, please give details:
                          Date   Results and comments
Hearing   _____   _____
Sight   _____   _____

Has your child been seen professionally by anyone for speech and language? Yes ☐ No ☐
If yes,
Who: _____Where: _____When: _____

Did this lead to any treatment?   Yes ☐   No ☐
If yes, what, if any, activities were given to help your child's speech and language?

_____

What do you feel are some reasons for your child's speech or language delay?

_____

_____

Do you feel your child has any other problems that affect speech or language development?

_____

_____

Would you like your child to improve in any of the following skills? Please tick.

Skills	Yes (tick)	Comments
Eating		
Drinking		
Toileting		
Walking		
Using hands		
Attending		
Listening		
Playing		
Talking		
Understanding speech		
Following directions		
Behaviour		
Getting along with other children		
Other (please specify)		

What aspects of your child's development are you most worried about?

_____

_____

How well do you think your child will communicate eventually?

_____

_____

During the past six months, have these skills changed? Is it noticeable that they are more, about the same or less? Please tick.

Skills	More	About the same	Less	Comments
Sounds				
Gestures				
Words				
Asking questions				
Using actions or gestures to communicate				
Understanding speech				
Talking to self				
Talking to others				
Playing alone				
Playing with others				

If your child talks, does he or she do any of the following:

Skills	Yes	No	Give example
Name people or things			
Ask for help, eg 'drink', 'wash dolly'			
Ask for information, e.g. 'what's that?' or 'where's bubba?'			
Imitate speech			
Call someone			
Greet someone			
Talk to self			
Give information, e.g. 'daddy home'			

What do you expect your child to do next in his or her communication development?

_____

_____

Are you doing anything special at present to help your child to communicate better? If yes, please give details

_____

_____

What kind of help, if any, do you want for your child at the moment?

_____

_____

Is there anything else you would like to tell us about your child?

_____

_____

Observation tasks

Now look at some of the skills that help children to learn to talk. Play with your child and see what he does. Choose a time when you both feel good and are ready to play together. Use toys or books that you know the child enjoys. Follow his lead. Talk about what you are both doing. There is no need to complete all sections of the observation task in the one session.

Looking together and attending

Use three objects that the child knows, such as a soft toy, small car or ball. Show them to the child, one by one. Let the child touch or play with each one after looking at it. Which objects did the child look at and approximately for how long (in seconds) did he play with each object?

Did the child look at it?

Object	Yes	No	How long (seconds)?
1.			
2.			
3.			

Appropriate play

Play with your child for at least five minutes with three familiar toys or objects. If necessary, show your child how to play with the toys. As you play, watch the way he plays with the toys. Be sure you select toys or objects that your child has already played with or seen.

Toy or object	What did child do?	Comment
1.		
2.		
3.		

Early intentional communication with another person

While the child is playing with one of the toys, move it so that the child can see it but cannot reach it. Record any action, gesture, sound or word he uses to protest and or ask for the toy to be returned.

Toy or object	What did child do or say	Comment

Now introduce a new toy or object that you know the child really likes, holding or placing it just out of reach. Record any action, gesture, sound or word the child uses to indicate that he or she would like to have it.

Toy or object	What did child do or say	Comment

Imitating actions

Using toys and objects that the child is familiar with, such as a car, ball, spoon and cup or a doll, choose some actions that you know he can do, such as pushing the car, rolling the ball or feeding the doll. Make sure the child is watching as you do each of the actions and encourage the child to imitate you. Say 'Do this' or '. . . (child's name), do this'. Praise the child if he or she imitates your action.

Action	Did the child imitate you?	Yes	Almost	No	Comment
1.					
2.					
3.					

Imitating sounds

Select three sounds you have heard the child make. When your child is watching you, make each of the sounds and encourage imitation. Encourage the child to look at you and say, for example, '. . . (child's name), say ba'. Model each sound no more than three times.

Sounds	Did the child imitate you?	Yes	Almost	No	Comment
1.					
2.					
3.					

Imitating words

Show the child three familiar objects that you know the child can name, such as a cup, an apple or a ball. Encourage the child to look at you or the object and imitate you when you label each object. Encourage the child to imitate the name of the object. Say '. . . (child's name), say ball'. Model each word no more than three times.

Words	Did the child imitate you?	Yes	Almost	No	Comment
1.					
2.					
3.					

Understanding object labels

Find three objects that are very familiar to the child, such as a soft toy, a hat or a book. Encourage the child to touch, point or in some way show you each object as you name it. Say '. . . (child's name), show me teddy'. Give the child no more than three opportunities to show you that he or she understands the object labels.

Object label	What did the child do?	Comment
1.		
2.		
3.		

Understanding action words

Find three objects that you know are familiar to your child, such as a car, a soft toy and a teapot and cup. Ask him to show you what to do with the objects. Say 'Show me how the car goes', 'Show me how teddy walks' and 'Show me how you pour some tea'.

What did you say?	What did child do?	Comment
1.		
2.		
3.		

Following directions

Find three objects that are familiar to the child. Select an action for him or her to carry out with each object. Choose actions that you know he or she understands and can do. Ask the child to do each action. For example, 'show me how you kiss dolly', 'show me how you put the car in the box', 'show me how you brush hair'.

What did you say?	What did the child do?	Comment
1.		
2.		
3.		

Using language

Play with your child using the same objects you selected to answer the previous questions. Now do the following tasks:

Object labels

Ask the child to name the objects you are playing with.

Object	What did the child say?	Comment
1.		
2.		
3.		

Action words

Ask the child to tell you what is happening when you do something with the toys you are playing with. Say 'what's happening?', while you make the dolly walk, kiss the teddy or drink from the cup.

Action	What did the child say?	Comment
1.		
2.		
3.		

Now make a list of the gestures, sounds and words used by your child to communicate while you played together. Write these down on the 'Sounds, gestures, words or phrases' communication record form (Appendix C).

Index